Wounds and Wound Management

Guest Editor

MICHAEL D. CALDWELL, MD, PhD

SURGICAL CLINICS
OF NORTH AMERICA

www.surgical.theclinics.com

Consulting Editor
RONALD F. MARTIN, MD

December 2010 • Volume 90 • Number 6

SAUNDERS an imprint of ELSEVIER, Inc.

W.B. SAUNDERS COMPANY

A Division of Elsevier Inc.

1600 John F. Kennedy Blvd., Suite 1800, Philadelphia, PA 19103-2899

http://www.theclinics.com

SURGICAL CLINICS OF NORTH AMERICA Volume 90, Number 6
December 2010 ISSN 0039–6109, ISBN-13: 978-1-4377-2616-9

Editor: John Vassallo, j.vassallo@elsevier.com

Developmental Editor: Jessica Demetriou

Surgical Clinics of North America (ISSN 0039–6109) is published bimonthly by Elsevier Inc., 360 Park Avenue South, New York, NY 10010-1710. Months of publication are February, April, June, August, October, and December. Business and Editorial Offices: 1600 John F. Kennedy Blvd., Suite 1800, Philadelphia, PA 19103-2899. Periodicals postage paid at New York, NY and additional mailing offices. Subscription prices are $311.00 per year for US individuals, $532.00 per year for US institutions, $152.00 per year for US students and residents, $381.00 per year for Canadian individuals, $661.00 per year for Canadian institutions, $429.00 for international individuals, $661.00 per year for international institutions and $210.00 per year for Canadian and foreign students/residents. To receive student/resident rate, orders must be accompanied by name of affiliated institution, date of term, and the *signature* of program/residency coordinator on institution letterhead. Orders will be billed at individual rate until proof of status is received. Foreign air speed delivery is included in all *Clinics* subscription prices. All prices are subject to change without notice. POSTMASTER: Send address changes to *Surgical Clinics*, Elsevier Health Sciences Division, Subscription Customer Service, 3251 Riverport Lane, Maryland Heights, MO 63043. **Customer Service (orders, claims, online, change of address): Telephone: 1-800-654-2452 (U.S. and Canada); 314-447-8871 (outside U.S. and Canada). Fax: 314-447-8029. E-mail: journalscustomerservice-usa@elsevier.com (for print support); journalsonline support-usa@elsevier.com (for online support).**

Reprints. For copies of 100 or more, of articles in this publication, please contact the Commercial Reprints Department, Elsevier Inc., 360 Park Avenue South, New York, New York 10010-1710. Tel. (212) 633-3812, Fax: (212) 462-1935, e-mail: reprints@elsevier.com.

The Surgical Clinics of North America is also published in Spanish by McGraw-Hill Interamericana Editores S.A., P.O. Box 5-237 06500 Mexico D.F. Mexico; and in Portuguese by Interlivros Edicoes Ltda., Rua Comandante Coelho 1085, CEP 21250, Rio de Janeiro, Brazil; and in Greek by Paschalidis Medical Publications, Athens Greece.

The Surgical Clinics of North America is covered in *MEDLINE/PubMed (Index Medicus)*, *EMBASE/Excerpta Medica*, *Current Contents/Clinical Medicine*, *Current Contents/Life Sciences*, *Science Citation Index*, and *ISI/BIOMED*.

Printed and bound by CPI Group (UK) Ltd, Croydon, CR0 4YY

Transferred to Digital Print 2012

Contributors

CONSULTING EDITOR

RONALD F. MARTIN, MD
Staff Surgeon, Department of Surgery, Marshfield Clinic, Marshfield, Wisconsin; Clinical Associate Professor, University of Wisconsin School of Medicine and Public Health, Madison, Wisconsin; Colonel, Medical Corps, United States Army Reserve

GUEST EDITOR

MICHAEL D. CALDWELL, MD, PhD, FACS
Department of Surgery, Marshfield Clinic, Marshfield, Wisconsin

AUTHORS

ADRIAN BARBUL, MD, FACS
Chief, Department of Surgery, Sinai Hospital of Baltimore; Johns Hopkins Medical Institutions, Baltimore, Maryland

CARRIE E. BLACK, MD
General Surgery Residency Program, Department of General Surgery, Marshfield Clinic, Marshfield, Wisconsin

MICHAEL D. CALDWELL, MD, PhD, FACS
Department of Surgery, Marshfield Clinic, Marshfield, Wisconsin

CAROL COPELAND, MD
Director of Orthopedic Trauma, Department of Orthopedic Surgery, Sinai Hospital of Baltimore, Baltimore, Maryland

J. WILLIAM COSTERTON, PhD
Director of Microbiology Research, Department of Orthopedic Surgery; Director of Biofilm Research, Allegheny-Singer Research Institute, Allegheny General Hospital, Pittsburgh, Pennsylvania

ROBERT F. DIEGELMANN, PhD
Professor of Biochemistry and Molecular Biology, Virginia Commonwealth University Medical Center, Richmond, Virginia

VINCENT FALANGA, MD, FACP
Department of Dermatology; NIH Center of Biomedical Research Excellence, Roger Williams Medical Center, Providence, Rhode Island; Departments of Dermatology and Biochemistry, Boston University School of Medicine, Boston, Massachusetts

STEPHANIE R. GOLDBERG, MD
Department of Surgery, Virginia Commonwealth University Medical Center, West Hospital, Richmond, Virginia

SHARON HENRY, MD, FACS
Chief, Division of Wound Healing and Metabolism, Department of Surgery, Shock Trauma Center, University of Maryland Medical Center, Baltimore, Maryland

SANDRA L. KAVALUKAS, PA-C
Department of Surgery, Sinai Hospital of Baltimore, Baltimore, Maryland

MARKÉTA LÍMOVÁ, MD
Clinical Professor, Department of Dermatology, University of California San Francisco, San Francisco; Private Practice, Fresno, California

SANJAY MUNIREDDY, MD
Department of Surgery, Sinai Hospital of Baltimore, Baltimore, Maryland

MICHAL NAWALANY, MD
Clinical Faculty, Department of Vascular Surgery, Marshfield Clinic, Marshfield, Wisconsin

JAYMIE PANUNCIALMAN, MD
Department of Dermatology; NIH Center of Biomedical Research Excellence, Roger Williams Medical Center, Providence, Rhode Island

HABEEBA PARK, MD
Resident, Department of Surgery, Sinai Hospital of Baltimore, Baltimore, Maryland

RONNIE WORD, MD
Department of Surgery, Marshfield Clinic, Marshfield, Wisconsin

Contents

The purpose of this article is to review the concepts behind, and practice of, wound surgery. The techniques of wound surgery, born of necessity in the art of military surgeons, have found their renaissance in the modern age of wound care driven by the economic and functional considerations inherent to the outcome-based management of chronic disease. Over 300 years of literature on wound healing has shown an innate ability of the wound (in the absence of infection and repeated trauma) to control its progress, largely through the local inflammatory cells. This article discusses several historical works on wound surgery and healing, topical wound therapy, minimal intervention, and emphasizes the closure of chronic wounds.

Surgeons often care for patients with conditions of abnormal wound healing, which include conditions of excessive wound healing, such as fibrosis, adhesions, and contractures, as well as conditions of inadequate wound healing, such as chronic nonhealing ulcers, recurrent hernias, and wound dehiscences. Despite many recent advances in the field, which have highlighted the importance of adjunct therapies in maximizing the healing potential, conditions of abnormal wound healing continue to cause significant cost, morbidity, and mortality. To understand how conditions of abnormal wound healing can be corrected, it is important to first understand the basic principles of wound healing.

Biofilms are a collection of microbes that adhere to surfaces by manufacturing a matrix that shields them from environmental elements. Wound biofilms are difficult to evaluate clinically, and standard culture methods are inadequate for capturing the true bioburden present in the biofilm. New molecular techniques provide the means for rapid detection and evaluation of wound biofilms, and may prove to be useful in the clinical setting. Studies have shown that many commercial topical agents and wound dressings in use are ineffective against the biofilm matrix. At this stage, mechanical debridement appears to be essential in the eradication of a wound biofilm. Topical antimicrobial agents and antibiotics may be effective in the treatment of the wound bed after debridement in the prevention of biofilm reformation.

Skin ulceration is a major source of morbidity and is often difficult to manage. Ulcers caused by an inflammatory cause or microvascular occlusion are particularly challenging in terms of diagnosis and treatment. The management of such ulcers requires careful assessment of associated systemic conditions and a thorough analysis of the ulcer's clinical and histologic findings. In this article, the authors discuss several examples of inflammatory ulcers and the approach to the diagnosis and treatment of these ulcers.

Complex wounds present a challenge to both the surgeon and patient in operative management, long-term care, cosmetic outcome, and effects on lifestyle, self-image, and general health. Each patient with complex wounds usually manifests multiple risk factors for their development. This article focuses on complex wounds involved with traumatic and orthopedic blunt or penetrating injuries, particularly in the extremities, as well as massive soft tissue infections including necrotizing fasciitis, gas gangrene, and Fournier gangrene. The principles of management of complex wounds involve assessing the patient's clinical status and the wound itself, appropriate timing of intervention, providing antibiotic therapy when necessary, and planning and executing surgical therapy, including the establishment of a clean wound bed and closure/reconstructive strategies.

Venous ulceration is the most serious consequence of chronic venous insufficiency. The disease has been known for more than 3.5 millennia with wound care centers established as early as 1500 bc. Unfortunately, still today it is a very poorly managed medical condition by most physicians despite that a great deal has been learned about the pathogenesis and treatment for venous ulcerations. We find that many wound care clinics treat the wound and not the cause of the problem. In this article, we review the basic pathophysiology of advanced chronic venous insufficiency and review the most up-to-date information with regard to medical therapy and different options of surgical therapy to address the underlying venous pathology responsible for chronic ulcers.

In recent years percutaneous therapy has gradually been adopted as an alternative to primary amputation in persons deemed unsuitable as surgical candidates, and has established itself as a primary mode of treatment.

There has been an explosion in endovascular technology and a revolution in revascularization patterns for limb salvage. Open surgery is now frequently reserved for failure of endovascular attempts or pathology unsuitable for endovascular revascularization. This article aims to educate the practicing general surgeon about the usefulness and appropriate application of different therapeutic endovascular options as applied to limb salvage.

The abdominal cavity represents one of the most active areas of surgical activity. Surgical procedures involving the gastrointestinal (GI) tract are among the most common procedures performed today. Healing of the GI tract after removal of a segment of bowel and healing of the peritoneal surfaces with subsequent adhesion formation remain vexing clinical problems. Interventions to modify both the responses are myriad, yet a full understanding of the pathophysiology of these responses remains elusive. Different aspects of GI and peritoneal healing, with associated factors, are discussed in this article.

Extensive skin loss and chronic wounds present a significant challenge to the clinician. With increased understanding of wound healing, cell biology, and cell culture techniques, various synthetic dressings and bioengineered skin substitutes have been developed. These materials can protect the wound, increase healing, provide overall wound coverage, and improve patient care. The ideal skin substitute may soon become a reality.

THE CLINICS ARE NOW AVAILABLE ONLINE!

Access your subscription at:
www.theclinics.com

Foreword

Wounds and Wound Healing

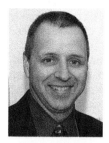

Ronald F. Martin, MD
Consulting Editor

The Accreditation Council for Graduate Medical Education (ACGME) released its final ruling on resident supervision and duty hour restrictions to be enacted 1 July 2011. The full report can be found on their website www.acgme.org. You have noticed that the topic of this issue of the *Surgical Clinics of North America* is about wound healing and you may be wondering what does the ACGME report have to do with wound healing. In a word—expectations.

Nearly everyone in the surgical education community within the United States has been grappling with the seemingly endless focus on work regulations for the past several years. This has been a contentious debate that has inflamed passions and been espoused by many groups with varying degrees of interest and self-interest. Many feel the science has been weak, although others argue to the contrary. Some argue that the proposed, now declared, changes are a political necessity to stave off some draconian action from without the body politic of medicine. There may be some truth to all or none of the above but, in my opinion, how true the claims are is more or less irrelevant as it misses the fundamental point: are we trying to manage expectations without regard to consequences?

A recent article in the *New York Times*, "What is it about 20-somethings?" by Robin Marantz Henig (18 August 2010), reviewed, among other things, some of the work of Dr Arnett on a phase of life he coined as "emergent adulthood." The article describes how the pursuit and achievement of many life goals for younger people have been delayed, or sometimes omitted, compared to similarly aged people in past times. The phenomena of young people graduating from college or graduate school to move back into their parents' homes and the longer period of time that parents provide tangible support for their adult children are discussed and a number of observations are relayed. Perhaps the question alluded to that intrigues me most is whether this phenomenon of delayed achievement of independence (for lack of a better

doi:10.1016/j.suc.2010.10.002
0039-6109/10/$ — see front matter © 2010 Elsevier Inc. All rights reserved.

surgical.theclinics.com

term) is causative of the prolongation of parental support or is the prolonged support of parents enabling the delay of, or even inhibiting, the younger person's development.

The fact that people tend to live longer than we used to is considered in this analysis of observed delayed maturation. It is suggested that perhaps it is a good thing for people to spend more time experimenting with options and exploring self-discovery before committing to a life course that will last longer than in previous eras. In many ways that seems reasonable. If one acknowledges even a fraction of truth in these observations, then perhaps we should seriously reconsider medical education and, in particular, surgical education—at least as far as expectations over time are concerned.

During the time that I have been involved in surgical education, there has been a steady decline in the amount of time that medical students were expected to spend "working" on their education and a concomitant decrease in the amount of responsibility that they should or could assume. Over that period of time I would submit that first day surgical residents have become progressively less able to function as effectively as their predecessors based on their preparation in medical school. Also, the curve of readiness of individual responsibility has been progressively been shifting toward the "right" of the timeline and now seems to spilling over into fellowship and junior attending. And maybe this is okay to a point, if it is a consensus change among those who need more time to train and those who expect a level of independent capability. My observation has been that no such pervasive agreement exists at present.

If the 20-somethings' general trend of a slower, more meandering path toward full development were a true cultural change, then this should probably apply to the group of people who we train as well. There is some age variance in the group of residents nationally, to be sure, but the concept probably still holds. If so, we as an organization had better address the changing dynamic while we can. Who knows, perhaps next year we'll hear about the 30-somethings that need more time to make it to 40.

The ACGME decision to limit the hours and opportunities for residents to learn, and redefining the work capacity of first year residents as a completely different kind of work schedule, much more akin to the current level of expectation of medical students, is a tacit declaration from our powers-that-be that these young persons are on a different path than those before. We have redefined the expectation of involvement without redefining the expectation of achievement. The amount and type of information they need to learn are not different. The amount of technical practice and clinical opportunities that are needed are no less than before, more likely they are greater than previously required. We are embarking on a path of changing expectations of effort, opportunity, and capacity without, in my opinion, proper regard to the consequences of altered training.

Perhaps we can work through this disconnect. We could lengthen training, uniformly disliked by trainers, trainees, and those who have to pay for it alike. We could modularize training and certification, problematic for historical reasons as well as its potential implications for existing organizations of considerable influence. We could separate the surgical education world from the rest of graduate medical education, although that would be a Herculean task with staunch opposition. Or perhaps we can ignore this while we produce trainees who are less confident and perhaps less competent as they enter practice.

Every cutting surgeon deals with wounds. Most wounds heal without significant post closure intervention from surgeons, at least, the simple ones. We have largely come to expect that time heals all wounds. Not so. For those wounds that do not heal well or present other challenges secondary to infection or host factors, changing our expectations or trying to limit the effort we will have to expend does not make them heal better. Wound healing is a complex biological process with multiple opportunities to not proceed the way we would hope—much like education. One big advantage when comparing wound healing to education is that we have reliable basic science to which we can turn and people who can put the science and clinical information in proper context. Dr Caldwell and his collaborators have assembled an excellent collection of articles to help us understand how wounds heal and how we can use that knowledge to impact outcomes positively. The information they have provided will help us reframe expectations of what we must do and how that will affect outcomes.

Last, Dr Caldwell and I would like to dedicate this issue to Dr Guido Majno. Dr Majno is a true pioneer of wound healing whose contributions to our understanding of the process and history of wound healing and inflammation are extraordinary. I first met him as a junior medical student when he was Professor and Chair of Pathology at the University of Massachusetts Medical School. He was one of those teachers whose impact lasted forever on all his students. We had hoped that he could have contributed to this issue but, unfortunately, because of health reasons he could not. In fact, he has contributed immensely to this issue throughout his life by all that we have learned from him. We wish him and his family the very best.

Ronald F. Martin, MD
Department of Surgery
Marshfield Clinic
1000 North Oak Avenue
Marshfield, WI 54449, USA

E-mail address:
martin.ronald@marshfieldclinic.org

Preface

Wounds and Wound Management

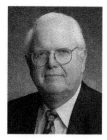

Michael D. Caldwell, MD, PhD
Guest Editor

This issue of *Surgical Clinics of North America* is designed to give the reader a summary of important concepts in wound healing. The authors have prepared excellent articles that range from the latest information in the basic science of repair to current techniques in difficult wound management.

I appreciate the opportunity to host this issue given to me by Ron Martin. I also greatly appreciate the contributions of each of the article authors and I hope that the reader will find their efforts to be as outstanding as I believe them to be.

We hope that this volume will provide the reader with new and intriguing knowledge of wounds and wound healing—and surgeons with an impetus to overcome the temptation of minimal intervention and actively engage in reducing the morbidity of chronic wounds.

Michael D. Caldwell, MD, PhD
Department of Surgery
Marshfield Clinic
1000 North Oak Avenue
Marshfield, WI 54449, USA

E-mail address:
Caldwell.Michael@mcrf.mfldclin.edu

Surg Clin N Am 90 (2010) xiii
doi:10.1016/j.suc.2010.10.001
0039-6109/10/$ — see front matter © 2010 Elsevier Inc. All rights reserved.

surgical.theclinics.com

Wound Surgery

Michael D. Caldwell, MD, PhD

KEYWORDS

- Vis medicatrix naturae • Wound • Debridement
- Delayed wound closure

"Je le pansay et Dieu le guarit."[1]
Ambrose Pare, AD 1885.

"The Chirurgion ought for the right cure of wounds to propose unto himselfe, the common and general indication: that is, the uniting of the divided parts, which indication in such a case is thought upon and knowne even by the vulgar: for that which is dis-joyned desires to bee united, because union is contrary to division."[1]

The loss of continuity of body substance by injury or disease was recognized by our ancestors as a painful, morbid, and frequently fatal process. Consequently, over the nearly 4 millennia of recorded medical history, physicians and surgeons have attempted by various means to speed the healing of wounds. The purpose of this introductory article is to review the concepts behind, and practice of, wound surgery. The techniques of wound surgery, born of necessity in the art of military surgeons, have found their renaissance in the modern age of wound care driven by the economic and functional considerations inherent to the outcome-based management of chronic disease. No longer allowed to rely largely on the "vis medicatrix naturae" dicta that populated minimal intervention-based wound care, modern wound care specialists our current are required to optimize all aspects of the wound bed and its closure.

VIS MEDICATRIX NATURAE AND THE BIOLOGIC PRIORITY OF HEALING WOUNDS

The term vis medicatrix naturae refers to the intrinsic healing power in a living organism, by virtue of which it can repair injuries inflicted on itself or resist disease. Although apparently wrongly attributed to Hippocrates, this phrase did encompass much of his philosophy toward the healing arts. One of the early writings relating this concept to wounds was by James Carrick Moore,[2] a member of the Surgeon's Company of London in 1789. In his dissertation Moore states: "When any accident or disease injures the human frame, it was early observed, that the body possessed within itself, a power of alleviating or remedying the evil. In consequence of this power it happens, that whenever the structure or functions of any part of the body are disturbed, such operations are immediately excited as have a tendency to restore the machine to its former state." In 1794, Hunter[3] concurred: "There is a circumstance attending accidental injury, which

Department of Surgery, Marshfield Clinic, WI, USA
E-mail address: Caldwell.Michael@mcrf.mfldclin.edu

Surg Clin N Am 90 (2010) 1125–1132
doi:10.1016/j.suc.2010.09.001
0039-6109/10/$ – see front matter © 2010 Elsevier Inc. All rights reserved.

surgical.theclinics.com

does not belong to disease-namely, that the injury done, has in all cases, a tendency to produce both the disposition and the means of cure." Moore[2] further concluded that inflammation is the process by which the vis medicatrix naturae fills wound cavities. Moore's dissertation was important in focusing the process of wound healing on local inflammation and the inflammatory cells. Unfortunately, as known by ancient surgeons, wounds exposed to air, along with many closed surgical wounds, suppurated. Thus, the mechanism by which inflammatory cells contributed to the healing process was obscured by the participation of these cells in abscess formation. In 1893, Lister[4] extended the earlier studies of Koch and Pasteur and demonstrated the evidence for bacterial growth in wounds and the ability of this growth to lead to abscess formation or invasive infection, sepsis, and gangrene. Lister's work to mitigate bacterial contamination led to important investigations into the basic elements of the repair process. For the first time, wounds could be examined in the absence of infection and the histologic response that interrelated inflammation and wound repair could be delineated. Therefore, the work of Virchow[5] was extended by Metchnikoff[6] and then subsequently by Stein and Levenson,[7] Simpson and Ross,[8] and Leibovich[9] to ultimately describe the central role of inflammation and inflammatory cells in tissue repair. Furthermore, by histologic observation, Metchnikoff[6] first introduced the concept of phenotypic interconversion between phagocytic and connective tissue cells. This concept was subsequently addressed by the work of Arlein and colleagues.[10] As summarized in a recent review, the finding of Moore that inflammation is the process by which the vis medicatrix naturae fills up cavities has come full circle and much of this process can be attributed to the functions and secretions of wound-associated macrophages.[11]

Consistent with the intrinsic healing power of wounds was the concept of the biologic priority of healing wounds. The writings of Virchow[7] described wound healing as a part of his discussion on the influence of blood vessels on local nutrition. He related that there was not only an increase in blood flow to an area of inflammation but also an increase in the extraction of nutrients from the blood supply to the inflamed part. This concept of a priority of substrate use by an injured or inflamed tissue was best enunciated by Moore.[12] Moore's concept was that because most wounds heal, even in the face of preinjury and/or postinjury starvation, there must be a biologic priority of a healing wound. Moore and Brennan[13] further proposed that: "The general biochemistry of injury and convalescence and the local changes of wound healing are in a sense two biochemical partners." These two biochemical processes maintained the mobilization of lean body mass after injury and increased the substrate pool available to the wound so that "the internal balance of the wound is positive, while for most other cellular tissues—particularly muscle and fat—it is negative."[13] Although the hormonal response to injury results in mobilization of body composition extraneous to the wound, wound metabolism seems much less responsive to circulating hormonal changes and more related to the metabolism of the wound's inflammatory cellular infiltrate.[14] Thus, at this juncture, over 300 years of literature on wound healing has shown an innate ability of the wound (in the absence of infection and repeated trauma) to control its progress, largely through the local inflammatory cells.

MINIMAL INTERVENTION IN WOUND CARE

The concept of minimal intervention in healing wounds, dates back to the earliest cuneiform writings in Mesopotamia,[15] and confirmed in the Edwin Smith surgical papyrus[16] and is reiterated in many of the writings of military surgeons. Thus, wound cleansing, topical wound therapy, and bandaging became the mainstay of wound care for almost 5000 years. Most surgeons attribute the basic principles of wound care to Ambrose

Pare's[1] The Apologie and Treatise in 1585. However, Pare properly attributes the origin of these principles to Guy de Chauliac, one of the most honored surgeons of all times. In his treatise, On Wounds and Fractures taken from the first important and complete work on surgery written in Europe in 1363, Guy de Chauliac prescribes the treatment of wounds. The treatment is "first, by Nature as the principal worker, which operates by its own powers and by suitable nourishment; and secondly, by the physician as a servant working with the five objects which are subalternate one to the other.

The first object requires the removal of foreign substances, if there are any such among the divided parts.

The second is to approximate the separated parts to each other.

The third is to preserve the parts thus brought together in their proper form.

The fourth to conserve and preserve the substance of the organ.

The fifth teaches how to correct complications."[17]

Pare[1] added to these concepts the use of gentle treatment and bland applications to wounds, replacing the boiling oil of the day.

TOPICAL WOUND THERAPY

It was not until approximately AD 25 that the cardinal signs of inflammation were described by Celsus. Erythema and swelling with heat and pain occur after all wounds; however, the earliest surgeons recognized that the survival of their patients was related to the character of the discharge from their wounds. If the cardinal signs of inflammation were followed by a thick creamy discharge (localization of infection and abscess formation), the patient usually survived. If, however, the wound discharge was thin, watery, brown, and foul smelling (characteristic of invasive infection), the patient usually died. Thus, suppuration was good (even laudable) and it led to granulation tissue formation and ultimately the healing of wounds. As a consequence, the historical treatment of wounds was based on methods that led to suppuration and involved techniques that controlled and localized the progress of wound infection. This empirical treatment worked even though the cause of the process was not clearly understood until late in the nineteenth century. The Edwin Smith surgical papyrus describes such topical therapy for wounds, dating from 1650 BC. Lint was used to promote capillary action and to pack and fill the wound space. Grease or oil was used because it did not spoil and decreased adherence of bandages to the wound. Honey was also used as a standard part of ancient topical wound therapy. Honey has been shown to have antibacterial properties that are thought to be because of both its osmolality and glucose oxidase content. The enzymatic action of glucose oxidase on glucose and molecular oxygen leads to the production of hydrogen peroxide. In addition to honey, lint, and oil (or grease), it was also common to use vinegar and wine for topical wound therapy. Wine has profound antibacterial properties out of proportion to its alcohol content. The antibacterial properties have been attributed to the presence of oenosides (polyphenolic compounds), which have been shown to be more than 30 times more potent than phenol in their antibacterial effects.[15,18] The ancient topical wound therapy frequently used metallic salts. The combination of metallic copper with acetic acid (easily found as vinegar in topical therapy) produces copper acetate, which has substantial antibacterial effects.[15] Therefore, the ancient surgeons, without fully understanding the rationale, developed techniques that allowed localization of infection through cleansing and bandaging of wounds and used topical compounds with antibacterial effects that led to laudable suppuration after inflammation, thus ensuring the survival of their patients. **Table 1** lists topical agents of wound therapy used by many of the more prominent surgeons

Table 1	
Historical aspects of topical wound agents	
Agents Used	**Surgeon**
Olive oil, honeycomb, gum arabic, incense	Johannes DeKetham, 1491
Zinc ointments, alum, sal ammoniac, turpentine	John Bell, 1810
Oil or wax, honey, copper sulfate, mercurial salts	Dominique Jean Larrey, 1814
Wine, lead acetate	Astley Cooper, 1825
Zinc sulfate, lead acetate, copper acetate, mercuric chloride	James Syme, 1832
Mercuric chloride, ammonium chloride, mercury and zinc cyanide, antiseptic treatment	Joseph Lister, 1884–1889
Sodium hypochlorite, epicutaneous treatment	Alexis Carrell, 1910
Silver foil, mercuric chloride, sodium hypochlorite	William Halsted, 1883–1917
Sulfonamide, penicillin, sodium hypochlorite, allantoin	Hamilton Bailey, 1947
Sulfonamide, penicillin, acetic acid	George Crile, 1947

in history. It is obvious from this table that empirical therapy present for a millennia was in common use until the work of Lister[19] in 1881. Lister's writings led not only to the aseptic protection of surgical wounds but also to the use of antibiotics directed at organisms that colonized or infected wounds.[19] Recent research has demonstrated that the success of topical antimicrobial agents is also dependent on adequate wound debridement to rid the wound of the microbial ecologic conditions that are characteristic of biofilms.

WOUND BED PREPARATION

The concept of wound bed preparation, which originated from the classical principles of Guy de Chauliac and Pare,[17,1] became refined with the organized, multidisciplinary approach to wound healing developed during the 1980s.[20,21] Wound bed preparation included debridement of nonviable tissue and denatured extracellular matrix, control of bacterial burden and inflammation, establishment of optimal moisture balance, and stimulation of epidermal cell migration of the wound edge and it subsequently became popularized under the acronym TIME.[22,23] The T referring to the removal of nonviable tissue, I to the control of infection and reduction of the bacterial burden, M to the maintenance of a moisture balance, and E to dealing with the advancing wound edge. Wound bed preparation is now established as a systematic approach for managing all types of chronic wounds.[23]

In acute wounds, debridement is used to remove devitalized damaged tissue and bacteria. Once this has been accomplished and any underlying comorbidities have been addressed, the clean acute wound bed usually heals readily. Chronic wounds, however, do not have the normal progression of inflammatory cells, accumulate proteolytic enzymes and abnormal cells that reduce the response to local peptide growth factors, and impede the growth of healthier cells. Thus, frequent debridement may be required to remove debris, wound exudate, and bacterial biofilms and thereby reduce bacterial bioburden.[24] The term chronic is generally used to refer to wounds that have not healed in 6 weeks. All chronic wounds begin as acute wounds; however, the patient's comorbidities, medications, environment, and behavior collaborate to alter the molecular and cellular environment of the wound and thus impaired healing.

Wound debridement serves multiple purposes: removes necrotic tissue that may nourish bacterial growth, removes pockets of infection, directly removes bacteria from the wound surface along with the biofilm critical for microbial ecology, removes desiccated tissue that interferes with cellular migration, removes senescent cells, and generally converts the wound bed to that found in an acute wound.[25] Debridement can thereby reinitiate the healing process. As stated earlier, the concomitant comorbidities must be addressed to optimize the benefits of surgical wound debridement. Arterial or venous insufficiency, trauma, blood loss, and edema all interfere with tissue perfusion and increase the likelihood of microbial proliferation. Adequate tissue perfusion allows oxygen, nutrients, and cells to be delivered to the wound and limits microbial growth.

An overlooked consideration in modern surgical wound debridement has been a mechanism for the accurate description, communication, and documentation of the process. The term debridement has been used without qualification or quantification. Recently, the International Advisory Board of Surgical Wound Management has put forward a mechanism to codify debridement practices. A descriptive classification similar to that used in oncological surgical resections was proposed in 2006.[26] Based on this classification, debridement is classified into 5 numerical categories: nondebrided wound (0), incomplete (1), marginal (2), complete (3), or radical (4). The nondebrided wound has not undergone the TIME-based wound bed preparation.[23] Incomplete debridement describes a process in which all nonviable necrotic tissue present at the time of debridement was not removed. Thus, this wound requires further debridement to optimize wound healing. Marginal debridement describes complete removal of all obvious necrotic nonviable tissue present at the time of surgery. Because some of the remaining tissue, although compromised, may be potentially viable, the marginal tissue has the potential to revive. In general, the more critical the tissue, the more likely the wound will not be initially debrided with the hope of revival on optimization of host comorbidities. This technique requires frequent observation and repetitive debridement. Complete debridement describes the complete removal of injured and infected tissue, both nonviable and potentially viable to the margin of normal tissue. This technique frequently necessitates serial debridements, after which, clear demarcation of normal tissue is evident. Recent innovations, such as the hydrodissection device, may achieve this state of debridement with fewer surgical procedures.[27] Radical debridement not only encompasses complete debridement but also includes a rim of clearly normal unaffected tissue. Thus, complete and radical debridements result in clean acute wounds, which is the goal of successful surgical wound bed preparation.

In recording the procedure, the lowest known category is chosen if there is indecision as to the extent of debridement.

In addition to describing the extent of tissue debridement, it is also important to know the type of tissue removed. The affected tissue can be allocated into 1 or more of the following 4 groups: skin (S), subcutaneous connective tissue (C) (consisting of fat, vessels, and nerves), deep soft tissue (M) (consisting of muscle, fascia, tendon, and periosteum), and bone (B). These categories further facilitate the communication and documentation of debridement without the use of less descriptive verbiage. By using this alphanumeric classification system, wound debridement can be thoroughly categorized and appropriately communicated.[16,26]

WOUND CLOSURE

Ancient surgeons observed that injuries with their margins in direct contact adhered and healed in a process described as healing by primary intention. Those wounds that lacked the necessary contact between the margins or succumbed to complications were mended by another process referred to as healing by secondary intention. The historical development of surgical techniques for the treatment of wounds reflected the efforts of surgeons to induce healing by the primary intention and remains the basis of wound and reconstructive surgery. Although Majno[15] relates that the art of sewing was known to the Neanderthals, as demonstrated by the clothing they constructed, the first recording of the suturing of wounds is found in case 10 of the Edwin Smith papyrus written between 2600 and 2200 BC. In his treatise Sushruta Samhita (between 1000 and 600 BC), Susruta suggested the use of cotton thread, hemp, leather, horsehair, and animal tendons to approximate the margins of wounds.[28] The hippocratic position regarding suturing was cautious. However, the technique is mentioned in the context of injuries to the face, nose, and lips.[29] Celsus described suturing of wounds at length. He reiterated the importance of cleansing and debriding the wound of all extraneous matter before suturing.[30] Owing to his firsthand experience in the treatment of the wounds of gladiators, Galen, like Hippocrates and Celsus, recommended the removal of all debris, cleansing of wounds, and early suturing.[30] Thus, by the second century AD, suturing of wounds was a common occurrence. In subsequent history, surgical and traumatic wounds were either sutured and healed by primary intention or healed by the lengthy process of secondary intention if the complications or surgical judgment did not allow the former.

CHRONIC WOUNDS: A CALL FOR CLOSURE

To quote Hampton[31]: "The basic objectives of wound management are to prevent or cut short infection in contaminated wounds, to eliminate the septic process in already infected and suppurating wounds, and in each to obtain sound healing. Surgical treatment of such wounds is designed to achieve these objectives with a maximum preservation of tissue, a minimum of scar, and a maximum return of function of the part in a minimum of time." Despite the evolution in suturing and wound closure techniques, including skin grafting and flap surgery (as reviewed by Santoni-Rugiu and Sykes[30]), the care of chronic wounds has not stressed the urgent need for surgical closure where feasible. The military experience in the World Wars I and II taught surgeons a new technique known variably as delayed primary intention, secondary closure, tertiary intention, or more properly, delayed suture or delayed closure.[32–35] This approach was popularized for civilian practice by Howe,[36] who recommended delayed closure for reopened postoperative incisional abscesses. The approach was further standardized by Robson and colleagues[37] based on bacterial quantification of the wound.

Another paradigm shift occurred in surgical wound care with the introduction of early tangential excision of burns by Janzekovic.[38] This technique removed necrotic tissue while preserving as much of the underlying viable tissue as possible, the hallmark of successful wound debridement. The wounds were then covered immediately with split-thickness skin grafts. When performed early, excision and immediate wound closure improved survival and decreased length of hospital stay.

Despite the significance of the contributions of delayed closure, and tangential excision with immediate skin grafting to surgical wound care, these modalities have not been universally included in the care of chronic wounds. It is the author's contention that the time has come for the renaissance of Hampton's 1954 dictum: "Every open wound needs and deserves surgery. Either it is ready for closure by suture or skin graft or it needs debridement to prevent or eliminate sepsis and the destruction of living tissue and to prepare it for closure...." Wound healing is a natural cellular process, provided the wound does not contain dead tissue, strangulated ligatures, or foreign bodies. Adequate surgery eliminates or prevents such particles and promotes early healing of the wounds, thereby achieving the objectives of wound management.[30]

It is hoped that this brief discussion and entreaty provides surgeons with an impetus to overcome the temptation of minimal intervention and encourages their active participation in reducing the morbidity of chronic wounds.

REFERENCES

1. Pare A. The apologie and treatise 1585. London: Falcon Educational Books; 1951. p. 122.
2. JC Moore. A dissertation on the process of nature in the filling up of cavities, healing of wounds, and restoring parts which have been destroyed in the human body. John Richardson printer to the Lyceum Medicum Londinense; 1789.
3. Hunter J. Treatise on the blood, inflammation and gunshot wounds. London: John Richardson Publisher; 1794. p. 190.
4. Lister J. An address on the aseptic management of wounds. Br Med J 1893; 161(1):277, 337, (subsequent correction).
5. Virchow R. Cellular pathology [Chance F, Trans; 2nd edition]. London: John Churchill; 1860. p. 283–315.
6. Metchnikoff E. Immunity in infective diseases [FG Binnie, Trans]. London: Cambridge University Press; 1905.
7. Stein JM, Levenson SM. Effect of the inflammatory reaction on subsequent wound healing in rats. Acta Chir Scand 1964;127:446, 125.
8. Simpson DM, Ross R. The neutrophilic leukocyte in wound repair. J Clin Invest 2009;51:1972, 106.
9. Leibovich SJ. The role of the macrophage in wound repair. Am J Pathol 1975;78:71.
10. Arlein WJ, Shearer JD, Caldwell MD. Continuity between wound macrophage and fibroblast phenotype: analysis of wound fibroblast phagocytosis. Am J Physiol 1998;275:R1041–8.
11. Rodero MP, Khosrotehrani K. Skin wound healing modulation by macrophages. Int J Exp Pathol 2010;3(7):643–53.
12. Moore FD. Metabolic care of the surgical patient. Philadelphia: WB Saunders Company; 1959. p. 58–9.
13. Moore FD, Brennan MF. Surgical injury: body composition, protein metabolism and neuroendocrinology. In: Ballinger, Collins, Drucker, et al, editors. Manual of surgical nutrition. Ballinger (TX): WB Saunders Co; 1975. p. 169–222.
14. Falcone PA, Caldwell MD. Wound metabolism. Clin Plast Surg 1990;17(3): 443–56.
15. Majno G. The healing hand: man and wound in the ancient world. Cambridge (MA): Harvard University Press; 1975. p. 37, 186–8, 115.
16. Breasted JH. The Edwin Smith surgical papyrus: hieroglyphic transliteration, translation and commentary V.1, Chicago: University of Chicago Press. Case 10, 1930. p. 226.
17. Chauliac Guy de. Inventorium sive collectorium in parte chirurgiciali medicine (or Chirurgia Magna) 1363. The section of wounds and fractures reprinted by the classics of surgery library. Birmingham (AL): Gryphon Editions, Inc; 1987. p. 17.
18. Ribereau-Gayon J, Peynaud E. Traite d'œnologie. Paris: Lib. Polytechnique Béranger; 1961. 124ff and 142.
19. Lister J. An address on the treatment of wounds. Lancet 1881;2(863):901.

20. Doucette MM, Fylling C, Knighton DR. Amputation prevention in a high-risk population through comprehensive wound-healing protocol. Arch Phys Med Rehabil 1989;70(10):780–5.

21. Knighton DR, Fiegel VD, Austin LL, et al. Classification and treatment of chronic nonhealing wounds. Ann Surg 1986;204(3):322–30.

22. Schultz GS, Sibbald RG, Falanga V, et al. Wound bed preparation: a systematic approach to wound management. Wound Repair Regen 2003;11(Suppl 1): S1–28.

23. Schultz GS, Mozingo D, Romanelli M, et al. Wound healing and TIME; new concepts and scientific applications. Wound Repair Regen 2005;13(Suppl 4): S1–11.

24. Falanga V. Wound bed preparation and the role of enzymes: a case for multiple actions of therapeutic agents. Wounds 2002;14:47–57.

25. Steed DL, Donohue D, Webster MW, et al. Effect of extensive debridement and treatment on the healing of diabetic foot ulcers. J Am Coll Surg 1996;183:64.

26. Granick MS, Chehade M. The evolution of surgical wound management: toward a common language. In: Granick MS, Gamelli RL, editors. Surgical wound healing and management. New York: London. Informa Healthcare; 2007. p. 17–27.

27. Granick MS, Jacoby M, Noruthun S. Efficacy and cost-effectiveness of the high-powered parallel waterjet for wound debridement. Wound Repair Regen 2006;14: 394–7.

28. Bhisagratna KK. The Sushruta Samita, English translation of the original Sanskrit. Text XI. The Chowkhamba Sanskrit Series, Varanasi (India). 1963.

29. Hippocrates. Hippocratic Writings. In: Lloyd GER, editor. Harmondsworth (NY): Penguin; 1978.

30. Santoni-Rugiu P, Sykes PJ. A history of plastic surgery. Heidelberg, New York. Berlin: Springer; 2007. p. 47.

31. Hampton OP. Fundamentals of surgery in contaminated and infected wounds. JAMA 1954;154(16):1326–8.

32. Ball WG. Lancet 1918;1:898.

33. MacPherson AIS. Delayed suture of soft tissue wounds. Lancet 1944;43–4.

34. Churchill ED. The surgical management of the wounded in the Mediterranean theater at the time of the fall of Rome. Ann Surg 1944;180(3):268–83.

35. Lowry KF, Curtis GM. Delayed suture in the management of wounds. Am J Surg 1950;280–7.

36. Howe CW. The early closure of constantly contaminated infected wounds with the aid of urethane-penicillin mixtures. Surg Gynecol Obstet 1948;87:425.

37. Robson MC, Shaw RC, Heggers JP. The reclosure of postoperative incisional abscesses based on bacterial quantification of the wound. Ann Surg 1970; 171(2):279–82.

38. Janzekovic Z. A new concept in early position and immediate grafting of burns. J Trauma 1970;10:1103–8.

Wound Healing Primer

Stephanie R. Goldberg, MD[a], Robert F. Diegelmann, PhD[b],*

KEYWORDS

- Acute wound • Phases of healing • Healing mechanisms
- Guidelines for healing

Surgeons often care for patients with conditions of abnormal wound healing, which include conditions of excessive wound healing, such as fibrosis, adhesions, and contractures, as well as conditions of inadequate wound healing, such as chronic non-healing ulcers, recurrent hernias, and wound dehiscences. Despite many recent advances in the field, which have highlighted the importance of adjunct therapies in maximizing the healing potential, such as optimization of nutrition, growth factor therapy, advanced wound dressing materials, and bioengineered skin substitutes, conditions of abnormal wound healing continue to cause significant cost, morbidity, and mortality. To understand how conditions of abnormal wound healing can be corrected, it is important to first understand the basic principles of wound healing.

PHASES OF WOUND HEALING

Wound healing consists of a complex but very orderly array of overlapping phases in which highly specialized cells interact with an extracellular matrix to lay down a new framework for tissue growth and repair.[1] There are 4 distinct but overlapping phases of wound healing, which include hemostasis, inflammation, proliferation, and remodeling (**Fig. 1**). These phases are influenced by the various cellular interactions and are regulated by the local release of chemical signals such as cytokines, chemokines, growth factors, and inhibitors.[2,3]

HEMOSTASIS PHASE

Immediately after tissue injury, hemostasis occurs to minimize hemorrhage. While the blood vessels constrict, platelets are activated by binding to the exposed collagen in the extracellular matrix. The platelets then release fibronectin, thrombospondin, sphingosine 1 phosphate, and von Willebrand factor, which promote further platelet

[a] Department of Surgery, Virginia Commonwealth University Medical Center, West Hospital, 16th Floor, West Wing, 1200 East Broad Street, Richmond, VA 23298-0645, USA
[b] Department of Biochemistry and Molecular Biology, Virginia Commonwealth University Medical Center, 1101 East Marshall Street, Sanger Hall, Room 2-007, Richmond, VA 23298-0614, USA
* Corresponding author.
E-mail address: rdiegelm@vcu.edu

Surg Clin N Am 90 (2010) 1133–1146
doi:10.1016/j.suc.2010.08.003
0039-6109/10/$ – see front matter © 2010 Elsevier Inc. All rights reserved.

surgical.theclinics.com

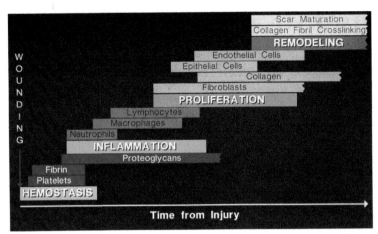

Fig. 1. Phases of normal wound healing. Cellular and molecular events during normal wound healing progress through 4 major integrated phases: hemostasis, inflammation, proliferation, and remodeling. (*From* Cohen IK, Diegelmann RF, Lindblad WJ, editors. Wound healing: biochemical and clinical aspects. Philadelphia: W.B. Saunders; 1993; with permission.)

activation and aggregation.[4] As these activation and other clotting factors are released, a fibrin matrix is deposited in the wound, which functions as a provisional matrix to stabilize the wound site. The aggregated platelets then become trapped in the fibrin matrix, thus forming a stable clot within the provisional matrix (**Fig. 2**).[5]

Several important mediators that are released by platelets are responsible for the initiation and progression of wounds through the subsequent phases of wound healing. These mediators include platelet-derived growth factor (PDGF) and transforming growth factor β (TGF-β). TGF-β and PDGF recruit additional cells, such as neutrophils and macrophages, to enter the wound. PDGF also recruits fibroblasts to the wound

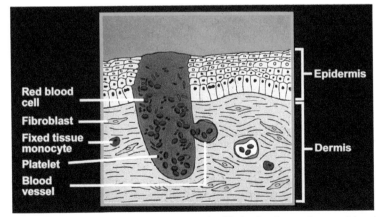

Fig. 2. Hemostasis phase. At the time of injury, the fibrin clot forms the provisional wound matrix and platelets release multiple growth factors that initiate the repair process. (*From* Greenfield, LJ, editor. Surgery: scientific principles and practice. Philadelphia: J.B. Lippincott, 1993; with permission.)

and activates the production of collagen and glycosaminoglycans by fibroblasts, which are important for the repair of the extracellular matrix.[2,3,6] Excessive levels of these growth factors have been indicated in conditions of abnormal wound healing; TGF-β is also present in many fibrotic conditions such as pulmonary fibrosis and cirrhosis.[7,8]

INFLAMMATORY PHASE

The next phase of wound healing is inflammation, which begins within the first 24 hours after an injury. The stage can last up to 2 weeks in patients whose wounds are healing appropriately but can last longer in those patients with chronic nonhealing wounds. From a clinical standpoint, this stage is characterized by rubor (redness), calor (heat), tumor (swelling), and dolor (pain), which results from the release of vaso-active amines and histamine-rich granules from the mast cells. These mast cell mediators cause surrounding vessels to become leaky and thus allow the efficient movement of neutrophils from the vasculature to the site of injury. Because the vessels become leaky, fluid also escapes into the area and thus causes the swelling (tumor) and pressure-causing pain (dolor).

In addition to mast cells, neutrophils and macrophages play key roles in the inflammatory phase (**Fig. 3**). Neutrophils serve as a first line of defense against infection by phagocytosing bacteria, damaged extracellular components, and foreign materials. As various chemical signals are released from the wound site, the endothelial cells in the nearby vessels are activated and begin to express specialized cell adhesion molecules (CAMs) called selectins. These CAMs function as molecular hooks to grab circulating neutrophils to bind to the endothelial cell surface by a process called pavementing. The adherent neutrophils begin to roll along the endothelial cell lining and then by a process called diapedesis, they squeeze through the cell junctions that have been made leaky by the mast cell mediators.[9,10]

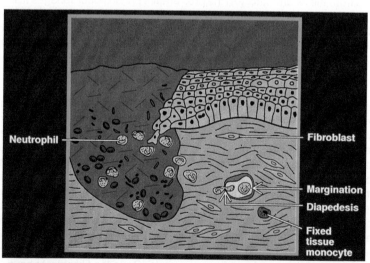

Fig. 3. Inflammatory phase. Within a day after injury, the inflammatory phase is initiated by neutrophils that attach to endothelial cells in the vessel walls surrounding the wound (margination), change shape and move through the cell junctions (diapedesis), and migrate to the wound site (chemotaxis). (*From* Greenfield, LJ, editor. Surgery: scientific principles and practice. Philadelphia: J.B. Lippincott, 1993; with permission.)

The neutrophils are attracted to the site of injury by a process called chemotaxis and are drawn there by soluble mediators, such as a breakdown product of a complement called C5a, a tripeptide f-Met-Leu-Phe (N-formyl-methionyl-leucyl-phenylalanine) that is a waste product produced by bacteria that may be present in the wound, and the potent chemokine interleukin (IL)-8.[11–13] To move through the extracellular matrix, the neutrophils release matrix-degrading enzymes, such as elastase and matrix metalloproteinase (MMP)-8, a collagenase. During a normal acute wound healing response, these enzymes are released in physiologic amounts and do not cause excessive tissue damage. In contrast, in many nonhealing chronic wounds, there is an overabundance of neutrophils, releasing massive amounts of these matrix-destroying enzymes that cause excessive damage to the extracellular matrix as well as the destruction of critical growth factors such as PDGF and TGF-β.[14–16] These ulcers are locked into a continuous inflammatory phase, resulting in extensive loss of tissue.[17]

On their arrival at the wound site, the neutrophils begin to aggressively phagocytize any foreign materials and kill bacteria by the powerful battery of enzymes and reactive oxygen species, which they can generate. The neutrophils actually initiate the first stages of the proliferative phase by releasing IL-1 and tumor necrosis factor (TNF)-α to begin the activation of fibroblasts and epithelial cells.

During the inflammatory phase, activated wound macrophages also play a key role in the regulation and progression of wound healing. Wound macrophages are derived from fixed tissue monocytes that originate from circulating monocytes (see **Fig. 3**). The wound macrophages are activated by chemokines, cytokines, growth factors, and soluble fragments of extracellular matrix components produced by proteolytic degradation of collagen and fibronectin.[18] The wound macrophages function to remove any residual bacteria, foreign bodies, and remaining necrotic tissue. The function of these macrophages is therefore similar to that of neutrophils, but macrophages better regulate proteolytic destruction of wound tissue by secreting protease inhibitors. In addition, macrophages ingest the bacteria-laden neutrophils and mediate progression of the wound from the inflammatory to the proliferative phase. Macrophages also secrete a multitude of growth factors and cytokines, such as PDGF, TGF-β, TNF-α, fibroblast growth factor (FGF), insulinlike growth factor 1, and IL-6, which then recruit fibroblasts and endothelial cells to the wound site for matrix deposition and neovascularization.

PROLIFERATIVE PHASE

The proliferative phase is characterized by fibroblast proliferation and collagen deposition to replace the provisional fibrin matrix and to provide a stable extracellular matrix at the wound site. The new matrix consists of collagen, proteoglycans, and fibronectins. In addition, angiogenesis occurs such that new blood vessels replace the previously damaged capillaries and provide nourishment for the matrix. Granulation tissue formation and the process of epithelization also occur.

Fibroblasts migrate into the wound in response to mediators released from the platelets and macrophages and move through the extracellular matrix by binding fibronectin, vitronectin, and fibrin via their RGD or arginine-glycine-aspartic acid amino acid sequence recognized by their integrin receptors (**Fig. 4**). The fibroblasts also secrete MMPs, which facilitate their movement through the matrix and help with the removal of damaged matrix components. Once the fibroblasts have entered the wound, they produce collagen, proteoglycans, and other components. Fibroblast activity is predominately regulated by PDGF and TGF-β. PDGF, secreted by platelets and macrophages, stimulates fibroblast proliferation, chemotaxis, and collagenase expression.

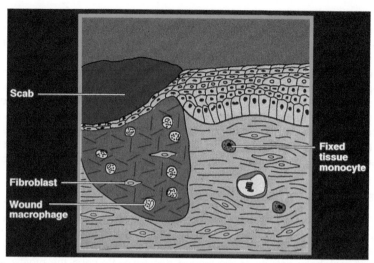

Fig. 4. Proliferation phase. Fixed tissue monocytes become activated, move into the site of injury, transform into activated wound macrophages that kill bacteria, release proteases that remove denatured extracellular matrix, and secrete growth factors that stimulate fibroblast, epidermal cells, and endothelial cells to proliferate and produce scar tissue. (*From* Greenfield, LJ, editor. Surgery: scientific principles and practice. Philadelphia: J.B. Lippincott, 1993; with permission.)

TGF-β has a central role in wound healing. There are 3 isoforms of TGF-β, which include TGF-β1, TGF-β2, and TGF-β3. TGF-β1 has been found to be present in excess amounts in conditions of fibrosis, such as pulmonary fibrosis and cirrhosis.[7,8] Although little is known about TGF-β2, TGF-β3 is associated with a reduction in fibrosis and scarring.[19] Despite their opposite effects on fibrosis, TGF-β2 and TGF-β3 bind the same TGF-β type 2 seronine/threonine kinase receptor, which then joins together with a TGF-β receptor (TBR) type 1 to activate the Smad cell signaling pathways.[20] Thus, activation of signaling cascades by the various TGF-β isoforms may account for the presence or lack of fibrosis within the wounds.

The most convincing studies that suggest a role for TGF-β in wound healing have been done in fetal animal models. Fetal mouse incisional wounds are known to heal without scarring and with a negligible amount of TGF-β present.[21,22] Lanning and colleagues[23] report that midgestational fetal wounds in the rabbit can be stimulated to contract in the presence of TGF-β1 and TGF-β3. In a study on the fetal mouse, rapid midgestational wound closure was associated with an increase in TGF-β1 and TBR-2 expressions compared with surrounding normal skin.[24]

Endothelial cells are activated by TNF-α and basic FGF (bFGF) to initiate angiogenesis such that new blood vessels are initiated to promote blood flow to support the high metabolic activity in the newly deposited tissue. Angiogenesis is regulated by a combination of local stimulatory factors, such as vascular endothelial cell growth factor (VEGF), and antiangiogenic factors, such as angiostatin, endostatin, thrombospondin, and pigment epithelium-derived growth factor. Local factors that stimulate angiogenesis include low oxygen tension, low pH, and high lactate levels.[25] Oxygen-sensing proteins regulate the transcription of angiogenic and antiangiogenic genes. Soluble mediators, such as bFGF, TGF-β, and VEGF, also stimulate endothelial cells to produce blood vessels. Tissue oxygen levels directly regulate angiogenesis through hypoxia inducible factor (HIF), which binds oxygen.[26] When there is a decrease in oxygen levels surrounding capillary endothelial cells, HIF-1 levels increase inside the cells and HIF-1 binds to specific DNA sequences to stimulate VEGF transcription to promote angiogenesis.

As the wound continues to heal, the granulation tissue forms to provide the transitional replacement for normal dermis and ultimately evolves into a scar. Granulation tissue consists of a dense network of blood vessels and capillaries, elevated cellular density of fibroblasts and macrophages, and randomly organized collagen fibers. The metabolic rate is also higher for this tissue compared with normal dermis, which reflects the activity required for cellular migration, division, and protein synthesis and thus, the importance of adequate nutrition and oxygen to properly heal the wound.

REMODELING PHASE

The last phase of wound healing is the remodeling phase in which granulation tissue matures into a scar (**Fig. 5**). Small capillaries aggregate into larger blood vessels and there is an overall decrease in the water content of the wound. Similarly, cell density and overall metabolic activity of the wound decrease. Perhaps the most dramatic change occurs in the overall type, amount, and organization of collagen fibers, resulting in increased tensile strength of the wound. Initially, there is increased deposition of type III collagen, also referred to as reticular collagen, that is gradually replaced by type I collagen, the dominant fibrillar collagen in skin.[27] Collagen fibers are cross-linked by the enzyme lysyl oxidase, which is secreted by fibroblasts in the extracellular matrix. As the wound continues to remodel, changes in collagen organization increases the tensile strength to a maximum of about 80% of normal tissue.

Extracellular zinc-dependent endopeptidases called MMPs have recently emerged as an exciting area in wound healing, which may have promising therapeutic potential. MMPs control the degradation of extracellular matrix components to facilitate epithelial cell migration into the wound, angiogenesis, and overall tissue remodeling. MMPs

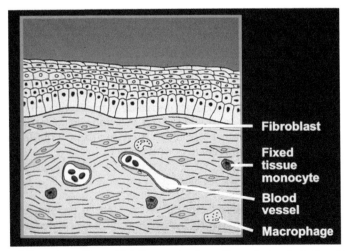

Fig. 5. Remodeling phase. The initial disorganized scar tissue is slowly replaced by a matrix that more closely resembles the organized extracellular matrix of normal skin. (*From* Greenfield, LJ, editor. Surgery: scientific principles and practice. Philadelphia: J.B. Lippincott, 1993; with permission.)

are secreted by epidermal cells and modulate tissue inhibitors of metalloproteinases (TIMPs) as well as degrade other growth factors.[28–31] Low levels of MMPs are found in normal tissue but increased levels of MMP-1 and MMP-2 are present in keloids, a condition of excess collagen deposition after cutaneous injury.[32] Similarly, a disruption in the balance between MMPs and their inhibitors has been reported in diabetic and venous stasis ulcers.[33,34] In addition, MMPs can be found in increased levels in chronic wounds.[35–38] Yager and colleagues[39] report that there are more than 10-fold higher levels of MMP-2 and 25-fold higher levels of MMP-9 in fluid from pressure ulcers compared with surgical wounds.

MMP expression is regulated by TGF-β. In normal fibroblasts and keratinocytes, abrogation of TGF-β1 is associated with decreased levels of MMPs and increased angiogenesis.[40–42] Tissue samples from keloids have demonstrated increased levels of MMP-2 and MMP-9 compared with healthy skin. Abrogation of TGF-β1 in keloid-derived fibroblasts results in a downregulation of MMP-9, further demonstrating the important relationship between TGF-β and MMPs.[43]

Treatment strategies targeted at the control of excess MMPs in chronic wounds have included the use of protease inhibitors to decrease MMP levels in the wounds and surrounding tissue. Oral and topical doxycycline, a potent MMP inhibitor, has been shown to decrease inflammation and matrix destruction.[44] Further studies are necessary to determine the clinical efficacy of doxycycline and other MMP inhibitors on chronic wounds.[45] TGF-β also minimizes matrix degradation by downregulating protease secretion and stimulating synthesis of TIMP.

As the extracellular matrix continues to remodel, collagen synthesis and degradation are ongoing as the matrix strives to achieve the original highly organized structure that was present before the wound injury. The scar tissue is always weaker than the normal surrounding matrix and can only achieve about 80% of the tensile strength that was present initially. If degradation maintains an equilibrium, then a fine line scar forms. If matrix synthesis is greater than degradation, then a hypertrophic scar may form. Conversely, if matrix degradation is greater than synthesis or if synthesis is inhibited by pharmacologic agents, such as steroids or cancer chemotherapeutic agents, or perhaps by malnutrition, the scar becomes too weak and wound dehiscence can occur.

MECHANISMS OF WOUND HEALING

Dermal wounds heal by 3 main mechanisms: connective tissue deposition, contraction, and epithelialization. Depending on the type of wound, these 3 distinct processes come into play to varying degrees. For example, an acute linear wound, such as a surgical incision that is closed by the surgeon using sutures, staples, tapes, or perhaps dermal glue, heals by what is termed primary intention. The major mechanism needed to heal wounds by primary intention is the process of connective tissue deposition. No contraction is needed because the surgeon has closed the incision by mechanical means. There is only minimal epithelization, which occurs along the wound line on the surface.

Open wounds, in which there is a loss of tissue, such as seen when a fingertip is injured, heal by a process termed secondary intention. These open wounds heal mainly by tissue contraction in which a centripetal force is generated by an interaction between fibroblasts and the matrix to advance the edges toward the center of the wound. There maybe some matrix deposition, and what is not achieved by those 2 processes is then covered by epithelization. Some chronic wounds, such as pressure ulcers, also heal by secondary intention once the chronic inflammation is controlled and granulation tissue is allowed to form.

If an open wound is suspected to be contaminated with foreign debris or bacteria, then the wound must be kept open and treated with gentle irrigation until the foreign materials and infectious agents are removed. As a general guide, the total bacterial burden should be lower than 10^5 organisms/g of tissue, as determined by biopsy and culturing.[46] Surface swabs are generally thought to be inaccurate. The wound should be gently irrigated with saline or lactated Ringer, and pressures greater than 15 psi should be avoided because they can force materials deeper into the wound bed and also damage newly forming granulation tissue.[47] Once these goals are achieved and if the wound can be closed, then the wound heals by a mechanism termed delayed primary intention.

Epithelialization is the process whereby epithelial cells surrounding the wound margin or in residual skin appendages, such as rete pegs, hair follicles, and sebaceous glands, migrate into the wound because of the loss of contact inhibition of cuboidal basal keratinocytes.[48] This type of healing is termed partial thickness healing and is observed in minor abrasions and skin graft donor sites when an approximately 0.015 in thick piece of skin is removed for coverage elsewhere on the patient. After an extensive multistep process, these basal epithelial cells proliferate near the wound margin, producing a monolayer that moves over the wound surface.

DEFINITION OF WOUNDS

For many years, lack of uniform definitions in the generalized description of wounds served as an impediment in setting forth guidelines for the treatment of wounds. In 1994, the Wound Healing Society sought to standardize the definitions of wounds and the evaluation of wound healing. A wound is defined as a disruption in the normal anatomic structure and function. Wounds can be classified as acute or chronic based on whether or not they progress through an orderly and timely healing process so as to restore anatomic continuity and function. Wounds are further differentiated based according to whether they are ideally healed, minimally healed, or acceptably healed based on various degrees of restoration of normal anatomy, function, structure, and appearance.[49] The problems associated with diabetic venous stasis and other complex and difficult wounds are addressed elsewhere in this issue.

GUIDELINES FOR THE HEALING OF ACUTE WOUNDS

The Wound Healing Society identified 11 categories of impediment to wound healing to formulate guidelines to promote the healing of acute wounds.[50] These include local impediments such as wound perfusion, tissue viability, hematoma and/or seroma, infection, and mechanical factors as well as systemic impediments that include immunologic factors, oncologic factors, miscellaneous systemic conditions, thermal injuries, external agents, and excessive scarring. The following summarizes the main clinical recommendations of the published guidelines.

Adequate blood supply must exist to provide oxygenation and nourishment to healing wounds, which can be maximized for elective surgical wounds by ruling out clinically significant arterial disease by the presence of palpable pulses or ankle-brachial indexes greater than 0.9, calculated as the ratio of the resting systolic pressure in the arteries of the ankle to that of the brachial artery. The lack of sufficient blood supply may lead to tissue ischemia and an increased risk of infection. Similarly, hypotension in the setting of acute wounds should be minimized. Patients should be advised to avoid smoking, blood glucose levels should be controlled, and hypothermia should be avoided, so to further maximize blood flow to the wounds.[51] The use of supplemental hyperbaric oxygen has long been thought to augment wound healing by increasing tissue oxygen levels; however, it has varied usage in the clinical setting. The Wound Healing Society guidelines suggest that more clinical data are necessary to support its use in acute wounds; however, a recent study demonstrated improved wound tissue oxygen tension in obese patients with supplemental oxygen administration.[52]

Wounds must be debrided of devitalized and infected tissue by one of the following methods, including preferably sharp surgical debridement and also enzymatic, mechanical, biologic or autolytic therapies. The formation of fluid collections, including hematomas, should be minimized by meticulous control of intraoperative hemostasis and correction of preoperative coagulopathies. Heparin prophylaxis against venous thromboembolism is indicated but may increase bleeding complications. There is no evidence according to the Wound Healing Society guidelines that antiplatelet agents increase the risk of hematomas. Similarly, the formation of seromas in patients with large skin flaps (mastectomy or component separation) should be minimized by closure of dead space and placement of surgical drains. The accumulation of fluid and blood may lead to local ischemia, necrosis, and an infected wound. Thus, postoperative fluid collections should be drained either surgically or percutaneously when possible.

Wounds should not be primarily closed if there is more than 10^5 bacteria/g of tissue or any amount of β-hemolytic streptococci because of an increased risk of wound infection.[46] A single dose of preoperative antibiotics is an indication in clean-contaminated or contaminated cases. Preoperative antibiotics are only recommended in clean cases if prosthetic materials, such as mesh, are implanted. Prophylactic antibiotics are not indicated in superficial nonbite injuries but should be used in bite injuries from animals and humans because they result in wound contamination. The risk of surgical site infections can further be decreased with normothermia and avoidance of hypoxia. Preoperative shaving of hair or scrubbing of the skin is not necessary to decrease the risk of infection because the bacterial load of normal skin flora is in the range of 10^3 organisms/g of tissue.

Wounds heal faster when closed primarily than those left to heal by secondary intention. Wounds should, however, be closed in a tension-free manner. Laparotomy incisions should be closed in a continuous manner using a suture length to wound length ratio of 4:1. The suture material used should be present until adequate tensile strength is obtained. The specific type of suture material used is irrelevant; however, permanent sutures are associated with an increased risk of fistulization. In patients with open abdomens, distractive forces that minimize subsequent fascial closure may be minimized through the use of negative pressure therapy. Retention sutures, long thought to be useful in preventing fascial dehiscence, do not prevent breakdown of the abdominal wall incisions.

Systemic immune defenses in patients with immune deficiencies should be maximized with the use of prophylaxis antibiotics, especially in patients with conditions such as AIDS. When possible, patients on immunosuppressants or steroid drugs should be weaned to the lowest possible dose preoperatively. Blood transfusions should be used with caution because they may result in transient immunosuppression.[53] Granulocyte-macrophage colony-stimulating growth factor may be used to correct leukopenia preoperatively so as to further maximize wound healing, but definitive studies have not been done to date.[54] In patients with cancer, operation performed through nonradiated tissue planes is associated with improved outcomes in wound healing. In addition, good nutrition is essential for optimal wound healing and can be augmented using preferably enteral means. Good nutrition is especially important in elderly patients and in those with cancer. Nutrition has traditionally been assessed by the measurement of prealbumin; however, this marker has proved to be unreliable in conditions of inflammation, acute renal failure, and corticosteroid use,[55] There are also insufficient data to support exogenous use of vitamins unless there is clear documentation of specific nutrient deficiencies such as those of vitamin C.

Burn injuries can be characterized as complex wounds consisting of shallow-partial thickness wounds, deep wounds, donor-site wounds resulting from skin graft harvest, or interstitial wounds from skin grafts. Each type of wound requires a different type of treatment. Partial-thickness wounds typically epithelialize within 21 days, whereas deeper wounds may require debridement of necrotic tissue with subsequent skin grafting for tissue coverage. Early debridement of deep burns has been advocated to minimize infection risk from necrotic tissue and promote normal healing, which has been associated with improved survivals. Permanent skin substitutes or temporary biologic or biosynthetic dressings may be used as an alternative to skin grafting should the excited burn total body surface area be too large to allow for donor grating. Deep wounds that cannot undergo early debridement may benefit from topical antibacterial agents; however, these agents have not been shown to be beneficial on shallow wounds, donor sites, or meshed skin grafts. There is no role for systemically administered antibiotics in the absence of systemic infection. The role of various vitamins and cofactors to augment wound healing is controversial. Zinc therapy may improve wound healing in zinc-deficient patients, yet routine use of zinc is not indicated. There are insufficient data to support the definitive use of vitamin C, vitamin E, and arginine. Pressure garments or compression dressings may be used to decrease fibrosis and scarring in burn injuries requiring more than 21 days to heal. Proliferative scars may benefit from silicone sheeting to decrease fibroblast activity and downregulate TGF-β. Direct injection of corticosteroids, including triamcinolone acetonide (Kenalog), may also improve proliferative scars. Postoperative radiation for benign conditions must be used with extreme caution; however, laser therapy may be useful.

Improved healing has not been seen in children or elderly with scald burns as well as in those with either inhalation injury or burns to the face and hands.

NORMAL AND PATHOLOGIC RESPONSES TO WOUND HEALING

Acute wounds progress through the phases in an orderly fashion for normal healing to occur. Chronic wounds begin the healing process in a similar fashion; however, they have prolonged inflammatory phase in which there is significant destruction of the matrix elements caused by the release of proteolytic enzymes from the neutrophils.[14–17] Once the excessive inflammation is controlled by aggressive wound care, then the proliferative and remodeling phases begin; however, the resulting scar is often excessive and fibrotic.[56] These chronic nonhealing ulcers are examples of severely deficient healing and are addressed in detail elsewhere in this issue. Despite extensive research into the mechanisms underlying wound healing, patients continue to be plagued by such pathologic conditions of abnormal wound healing in other tissues and organs, including recurrent and incisional hernias, anastomotic leaks, and wound dehiscence.

In conditions of fibrosis, the equilibrium between scar deposition and remodeling is such that an excessive amount of collagen deposition and organization occurs. This condition leads to a loss of both structure and function. Fibrosis, strictures, adhesions, keloids, hypertrophic scars, and contractures are examples of excessive pathologic healing.

Clinical differences between chronic and acute healing wounds are thought to be, in part, explained by alterations in the local biochemical environment. Acute wounds are associated with a greater mitogenic activity than chronic wounds.[57–59] Chronic wounds are associated with a higher level of proinflammatory cytokines than acute wounds. As chronic wounds begin to heal, they progress to a less proinflammatory state. Chronic wounds have elevated levels of MMPs compared with acute wounds.[16,39,56,60] Elevated protease activities in some chronic wounds may directly contribute to poor healing by degrading proteins necessary for normal wound healing, such as extracellular matrix proteins, growth factors, and protease inhibitors. Steed and colleagues[61] reported that extensive debridement of diabetic ulcers resulted in improved healing in patients treated with placebo or with recombinant human PDGF. Frequent debridement may therefore allow a chronic wound to heal in a similar fashion to an acute wound. In addition to the local wound environment, there are data to suggest that cells of chronic wounds may have an altered capacity by which to respond to various cytokines and growth factors and are in a senescent state.[62]

SUMMARY

The healing of surgical, acute, and chronic wounds requires the complex interaction of a multitude of cells, growth factors, and other proteins to allow the return of structure and function. Wound healing research only continues to evolve. With the creation of the Wound Healing Society guidelines as well as the significant contributions from researchers studying wound healing, the ability to modulate nonhealing wounds and facilitate wound closure continues to improve (http://www.woundheal.org).

REFERENCES

1. Diegelmann RF, Evans MC. Wound healing: an overview of acute, fibrotic and delayed healing. Front Biosci 2004;9:283–9.
2. Bennett NT, Schultz GS. Growth factors and wound healing: part II. Role in normal and chronic wound healing. Am J Surg 1993;166(1):74–81.
3. Bennett NT, Schultz GS. Growth factors and wound healing: biochemical properties of growth factors and their receptors. Am J Surg 1993;165(6):728–37.
4. Cho J, Mosher DF. Role of fibronectin assembly in platelet thrombus formation. J Thromb Haemost 2006;4(7):1461–9.
5. Gailit J, Clark RA. Wound repair in the context of extracellular matrix. Curr Opin Cell Biol 1994;6(5):717–25.
6. Rumalla VK, Borah GL. Cytokines, growth factors, and plastic surgery. Plast Reconstr Surg 2001;108(3):719–33.
7. Broekelmann TJ, Limper AH, Colby TV, et al. Transforming growth factor beta 1 is present at sites of extracellular matrix gene expression in human pulmonary fibrosis. Proc Natl Acad Sci U S A 1991;88(15):6642–6.
8. Gressner AM, Weiskirchen R, Breitkopf K, et al. Roles of TGF-beta in hepatic fibrosis. Front Biosci 2002;7:d793–807.
9. Frenette PS, Wagner DD. Adhesion molecules—part 1. N Engl J Med 1996;334(23):1526–9.
10. Frenette PS, Wagner DD. Adhesion molecules—part II: blood vessels and blood cells. N Engl J Med 1996;335(1):43–5.
11. Guo RF, Ward PA. Role of C5a in inflammatory responses. Annu Rev Immunol 2005;23:821–52.

12. Tschaikowsky K, Sittl R, Braun GG, et al. Increased fMet-Leu-Phe receptor expression and altered superoxide production of neutrophil granulocytes in septic and posttraumatic patients. Clin Investig 1993;72(1):18–25.

13. Roupe KM, Nybo M, Sjobring U, et al. Injury is a major inducer of epidermal innate immune responses during wound healing. J Invest Dermatol 2010; 130(4):1167–77.

14. Nwomeh BC, Liang HX, Cohen IK, et al. MMP-8 is the predominant collagenase in healing wounds and nonhealing ulcers. J Surg Res 1999;81(2):189–95.

15. Nwomeh BC, Liang HX, Diegelmann RF, et al. Dynamics of the matrix metalloproteinases MMP-1 and MMP-8 in acute open human dermal wounds. Wound Repair Regen 1998;6(2):127–34.

16. Yager DR, Chen SM, Ward S, et al. The ability of chronic wound fluids to degrade peptide growth factors is associated with increased levels of elastase activity and diminished levels of proteinase inhibitors. Wound Repair Regen 1997;5:23–32.

17. Diegelmann RF. Excessive neutrophils characterize chronic pressure ulcers. Wound Repair Regen 2003;11(6):490–5.

18. Diegelmann RF, Cohen IK, Kaplan AM. The role of macrophages in wound repair: a review. Plast Reconstr Surg 1981;68(1):107–13.

19. Shah M, Foreman DM, Ferguson MW. Neutralisation of TGF-beta 1 and TGF-beta 2 or exogenous addition of TGF-beta 3 to cutaneous rat wounds reduces scarring. J Cell Sci 1995;108(Pt 3):985–1002.

20. ten Dijke P, Hill CS. New insights into TGF-beta-Smad signaling. Trends Biochem Sci 2004;29(5):265–73.

21. Stelnicki EJ, Bullard KM, Harrison MR, et al. A new in vivo model for the study of fetal wound healing. Ann Plast Surg 1997;39(4):374–80.

22. Whitby DJ, Ferguson MW. Immunohistochemical localization of growth factors in fetal wound healing. Dev Biol 1991;147(1):207–15.

23. Lanning DA, Nwomeh BC, Montante SJ, et al. TGF-beta1 alters the healing of cutaneous fetal excisional wounds. J Pediatr Surg 1999;34(5):695–700.

24. Goldberg SR, McKinstry RP, Sykes V, et al. Rapid closure of midgestational excisional wounds in a fetal mouse model is associated with altered transforming growth factor-beta isoform and receptor expression. J Pediatr Surg 2007;42(6): 966–71 [discussion: 971–3].

25. Bhushan M, Young HS, Brenchley PE, et al. Recent advances in cutaneous angiogenesis. Br J Dermatol 2002;147(3):418–25.

26. Semenza GL. HIF-1 and tumor progression: pathophysiology and therapeutics. Trends Mol Med 2002;8(4 Suppl):S62–7.

27. Clore JN, Cohen IK, Diegelmann RF. Quantitation of collagen types I and III during wound healing in rat skin. Proc Soc Exp Biol Med 1979;161(3):337–40.

28. Chen WY, Rogers AA, Lydon MJ. Characterization of biologic properties of wound fluid collected during early stages of wound healing. J Invest Dermatol 1992; 99(5):559–64.

29. Vaalamo M, Leivo T, Saarialho-Kere U. Differential expression of tissue inhibitors of metalloproteinases (TIMP-1, -2, -3, and -4) in normal and aberrant wound healing. Hum Pathol 1999;30(7):795–802.

30. Trengove NJ, Stacey MC, MacAuley S, et al. Analysis of the acute and chronic wound environments: the role of proteases and their inhibitors. Wound Repair Regen 1999;7(6):442–52.

31. Singer AJ, Clark RA. Cutaneous wound healing. N Engl J Med 1999;341(10): 738–46.

32. Thielitz A, Vetter RW, Schultze B, et al. Inhibitors of dipeptidyl peptidase IV-like activity mediate antifibrotic effects in normal and keloid-derived skin fibroblasts. J Invest Dermatol 2008;128(4):855–66.

33. Cowin AJ, Hatzirodos N, Holding CA, et al. Effect of healing on the expression of transforming growth factor beta(s) and their receptors in chronic venous leg ulcers. J Invest Dermatol 2001;117(5):1282–9.

34. Galkowska H, Wojewodzka U, Olszewski WL. Chemokines, cytokines, and growth factors in keratinocytes and dermal endothelial cells in the margin of chronic diabetic foot ulcers. Wound Repair Regen 2006;14(5):558–65.

35. Wysocki AB. Fibronectin in acute and chronic wounds. J ET Nurs 1992;19(5): 166–70.

36. Wysocki AB, Staiano-Coico L, Grinnell F. Wound fluid from chronic leg ulcers contains elevated levels of metalloproteinases MMP-2 and MMP-9. J Invest Dermatol 1993;101(1):64–8.

37. Seah CC, Phillips TJ, Howard CE, et al. Chronic wound fluid suppresses proliferation of dermal fibroblasts through a Ras-mediated signaling pathway. J Invest Dermatol 2005;124(2):466–74.

38. Wysocki AB, Grinnell F. Fibronectin profiles in normal and chronic wound fluid. Lab Invest 1990;63(6):825–31.

39. Yager DR, Zhang LY, Liang HX, et al. Wound fluids from human pressure ulcers contain elevated matrix metalloproteinase levels and activity compared to surgical wound fluids. J Invest Dermatol 1996;107(5):743–8.

40. Philipp K, Riedel F, Germann G, et al. TGF-beta antisense oligonucleotides reduce mRNA expression of matrix metalloproteinases in cultured wound-healing-related cells. Int J Mol Med 2005;15(2):299–303.

41. Philipp K, Riedel F, Sauerbier M, et al. Targeting TGF-beta in human keratinocytes and its potential role in wound healing. Int J Mol Med 2004;14(4):589–93.

42. Riedel K, Riedel F, Goessler UR, et al. TGF-beta antisense therapy increases angiogenic potential in human keratinocytes in vitro. Arch Med Res 2007;38(1):45–51.

43. Sadick H, Herberger A, Riedel K, et al. TGF-beta1 antisense therapy modulates expression of matrix metalloproteinases in keloid-derived fibroblasts. Int J Mol Med 2008;22(1):55–60.

44. Golub LM, McNamara TF, Ryan ME, et al. Adjunctive treatment with subantimicrobial doses of doxycycline: effects on gingival fluid collagenase activity and attachment loss in adult periodontitis. J Clin Periodontol 2001;28(2):146–56.

45. Stechmiller J, Cowan L, Schultz G. The role of doxycycline as a matrix metalloproteinase inhibitor for the treatment of chronic wounds. Biol Res Nurs 2010;11(4): 336–44.

46. Robson MC, Mannari RJ, Smith PD, et al. Maintenance of wound bacterial balance. Am J Surg 1999;178(5):399–402.

47. Rodeheaver GT. Pressure ulcer debridement and cleansing: a review of current literature. Ostomy Wound Manage 1999;45(1A Suppl):80S–5S [quiz: 86S–7S].

48. O'Toole EA. Extracellular matrix and keratinocyte migration. Clin Exp Dermatol 2001;26(6):525–30.

49. Lazarus GS, Cooper DM, Knighton DR, et al. Definitions and guidelines for assessment of wounds and evaluation of healing. Wound Repair Regen 1994; 2(3):165–70.

50. Franz MG, Robson MC, Steed DL, et al. Guidelines to aid healing of acute wounds by decreasing impediments of healing. Wound Repair Regen 2008; 16(6):723–48.

51. Ueno C, Hunt TK, Hopf HW. Using physiology to improve surgical wound outcomes. Plast Reconstr Surg 2006;117(7 Suppl):59S–71S.
52. Kabon B, Rozum R, Marschalek C, et al. Supplemental postoperative oxygen and tissue oxygen tension in morbidly obese patients. Obes Surg 2010;20(7):885–94.
53. O'Mara MS, Hayetian F, Slater H, et al. Results of a protocol of transfusion threshold and surgical technique on transfusion requirements in burn patients. Burns 2005;31(5):558–61.
54. De Ugarte DA, Roberts RL, Lerdluedeeporn P, et al. Treatment of chronic wounds by local delivery of granulocyte-macrophage colony-stimulating factor in patients with neutrophil dysfunction. Pediatr Surg Int 2002;18(5–6):517–20.
55. Dennis RA, Johnson LE, Roberson PK, et al. Changes in prealbumin, nutrient intake, and systemic inflammation in elderly recuperative care patients. J Am Geriatr Soc 2008;56(7):1270–5.
56. Mast BA, Schultz GS. Interactions of cytokines, growth factors, and proteases in acute and chronic wounds. Wound Repair Regen 1996;4(4):411–20.
57. Bucalo B, Eaglstein WH, Falanga V. Inhibition of cell proliferation by chronic wound fluid. Wound Repair Regen 1993;1(3):181–6.
58. Katz MH, Alvarez AF, Kirsner RS, et al. Human wound fluid from acute wounds stimulates fibroblast and endothelial cell growth. J Am Acad Dermatol 1991; 25(6 Pt 1):1054–8.
59. Harris IR, Yee KC, Walters CE, et al. Cytokine and protease levels in healing and non-healing chronic venous leg ulcers. Exp Dermatol 1995;4(6):342–9.
60. Yager DR, Nwomeh BC. The proteolytic environment of chronic wounds. Wound Repair Regen 1999;7(6):433–41.
61. Steed DL, Donohoe D, Webster MW, et al. Effect of extensive debridement and treatment on the healing of diabetic foot ulcers. Diabetic Ulcer Study Group. J Am Coll Surg 1996;183(1):61–4.
62. Harding KG, Moore K, Phillips TJ. Wound chronicity and fibroblast senescence— implications for treatment. Int Wound J 2005;2(4):364–8.

Current Concepts Regarding the Effect of Wound Microbial Ecology and Biofilms on Wound Healing

Carrie E. Black, MD[a],*, J. William Costerton, PhD[b]

KEYWORDS

- Biofilm • Chronic wound • Microbiology • Microbial ecology
- Molecular diagnostics

A biofilm is an aggregation of microbes that manufacture a protective carbohydrate matrix, which allows them to adhere to each other and to a host wound surface. The matrix shields them from environmental factors that would otherwise lead to their eradication. Biofilms have been described as the predominant environment for most bacteria on the planet, and 99.9% of all microbial biomass on earth exists as a biofilm.[1] Biofilms are a primary source of contamination in a host of arenas from water treatment to medical prosthetic and catheter-related infections.[2,3] A commonly held belief has been that chronic wounds are caused by a single major pathogen and that polymicrobial growth represents colonization. However, biofilms by definition are polymicrobial, and due to their ability to share virulence factors, microbes form functional pathogroups within the biofilm.

ACUTE AND CHRONIC WOUNDS

Wounds are defined as chronic when they fail to progress through the expected trajectory of healing. Wound chronicity is loosely defined as a failure to heal after 30 to 60 days.[4,5] Acute and chronic wound healing can be immunohistologically differentiated by the unique set of immunoproteins present in each phase. In the acute wound, there is an upregulation of a nonspecific humoral response during the inflammatory phase

---

The authors have nothing to disclose.
[a] Department of General Surgery, General Surgery Residency Program, Marshfield Clinic, 1000 North Oak Avenue, Marshfield, WI 54449, USA
[b] Department of Orthopedic Surgery, Allegheny-Singer Research Institute, Allegheny General Hospital, 320 East North Avenue, Pittsburgh, PA 15212, USA
* Corresponding author.
E-mail address: black.carrie@marshfieldclinic.org

Surg Clin N Am 90 (2010) 1147–1160
doi:10.1016/j.suc.2010.08.009
0039-6109/10/$ – see front matter © 2010 Elsevier Inc. All rights reserved.

and the major cells present are polymorphonucleocytes (PMN), macrophages, and lymphocytes. In the chronic wound, there is an upregulation of matrix metalloproteinase (MMP) stimulated by cytokines, growth factors, and cell-cell contact, which impair wound healing. The factors responsible are specifically MMP 2, 8, and 9, tumor necrosis factor α, interleukin-1, and interferon γ. Bacteria present in the wound lead to disordered leukocyte function, poor angiogenesis and granulation tissue formation, and truncated wound contraction and epithelial migration. There is also stasis of cellular response seen in chronic wounds including a large number of neutrophils that release cytotoxic enzymes, free oxygen radicals, and other inflammatory mediators.[6–10] Biofilms are found in chronic wounds, and an estimated 60% to 80% of chronic wounds have biofilm present. Biofilms rarely exist on acute wounds because of the dynamic environment and interaction between host proteins and bacterial contamination. Thus the presence of biofilms forms a major difference between acute and chronic wounds. It has been postulated that certain cells upregulated in the chronic wounds prime the environment for biofilm formation. In animal models biofilm formation is rapid, and microcolonies are present within 8 to 10 hours after tissue injury in a controlled environment.[4,6,7,11,12]

INFECTION/COLONIZATION

The exploration of the molecular properties of biofilms over the last 3 decades has expanded our understanding of the chronic inflammatory process and the spectrum of colonization versus infection within wounded human tissue. A wound is considered infected by a live microbial cell count of greater than 10^5 organisms.[8,10,12] The pathway from colonization to clinical infection by an organism has previously been described as linear, defined by the total count of the live bacteria present in each phase. The understanding of biofilm complicates this simplistic view of the bacterial relationship with the host. A wound with a biofilm present does not show the clinical signs of acute infection traditionally defined by erythema, induration, and pain; yet in the biofilm the total count of live bacteria could exponentially exceed the standard for infection given above. Even though a biofilm within a wound does not elicit the typical host response, its presence requires intervention, because the host will not be able to overcome the biofilm without debridement.

BIOFILM MATRIX

The lifecycle of the biofilm can be described by stages of attachment, growth or maturation, and detachment. Understanding these stages, as well as the biofilm matrix, is essential for biofilm research and successful treatment.

Attachment

Attachment is regulated by specific cell surface receptors on the bacteria, which can sense an appropriate environment. This process can be categorized as docking and locking, a combination of physical and electrostatic interactions with adhesion molecules.[13] In particular, Heme protein and host extracellular epitopes cause the bacterial upregulation of adhesion proteins that bind collagen, fibrinogen, and fibronectin, thus converting the bacteria from planktonic to biofilm form.[8,9,14] As attachment occurs, protein expression of up to 50% of the bacterial proteome is changed, making the bacteria within a biofilm phenotypically different from their planktonic form. Microscopically, in conjunction with these changes the bacteria lose their mobility and begin to form cell clusters.[15]

Growth

The growth phase of the biofilm involves the synergistic ability of the bacteria from different species to work together to encase themselves in the carbohydrate matrix by quorum sensing. The bacteria become encased in a matrix that shows progressive cell layering, and the maximum average thickness of a mature biofilm has been found to be around 50 to 100 μm.[14,15] Quorum sensing also triggers efficient blood vessel invasion prior to biofilm formation following the increase in cell density. Factors contributing to biofilm growth are internal pH, oxygen perfusion, carbon source, and osmolarity.[13,16] When first discovered the biofilm was thought to be a static carbohydrate matrix, but further study has shown that it to be a widely dynamic environment. Organized into mounds and channels, the biofilm's topography has proven to be important in the transfer of exogenous solutes, nutrients, and oxygen.[17] The major source of nutrients for the bacteria within biofilm is not from devitalized tissue but from plasma and other exudates from the wound bed.[8]

Matrix

The biofilm matrix has been widely studied by light and electron microscopy. These techniques can demonstrate attachment within 5 hours, showing microcolonies with surrounding polysaccharide matrix, and within 10 hours the channels and mounds characterizing maturity are visible.[11,12] The extracellular polymeric substances (EPS) composing 80% of the biofilm consist of polysaccharides, alginate, extracellular DNA, proteins, and lipids.[8,10] This matrix is generally called the glycocalyx and is the distinguishing mark of biofilms.[13,18] The alginate in the matrix plays a particularly important role not only by providing structure but also acting as a scavenger of free O_2 radicals, preventing phagocytosis, and binding cationic antibiotics like aminoglycosides and tetracyclines.[10,11,13]

Detachment

In the initial studies on biofilm matrix, the detachment phase was considered passive by erosion and sloughing; however, this has also been shown to be an active process beginning from the structural hollow mounds with seeding dispersal of microcolonies and single cells in planktonic form.[2,15,17,19] Shedding and detachment have been shown in the research setting using direct visualization; however, it is still unclear to what degree the bacterial shedding from a biofilm contributes to the overall invasive microbial burden of a wound in the clinical setting.

BIO-ECOLOGY OF BIOFILM
Unique Physiology

The genetic profile and protein expression pattern of bacteria within a biofilm have been shown to be distinctly different from those of the same planktonic organisms. Oxygen only penetrates a few microns into the surface of biofilms, inducing adaptive responses such as anaerobic oxidation and iron-limitation stress for anaerobes and facultative aerobes. Although the distribution of the microcolonies of bacteria may at first glance appear to be random, studies have shown that certain species of bacteria are organized at specific depths of the biofilm, which may be related to specific physiologic properties at certain levels of the biofilm.[20,21] In addition, the protein RpoS, an adaptive stress protein, produced by *Escherichia coli*, which renders cells less vulnerable to pH, heat, or cold shock, has been found to be upregulated in high-density areas of the biofilm.[22,23]

Protein Upregulation

The ability of bacteria to participate in quorum sensing has been postulated to play a role in the genetic mutations that cause bacteria to transform into their biofilm form.[3,13,23] Iron is important in the quorum-sensing mechanism, and 44% of the genes involved in quorum-sensing regulation are induced in low iron conditions.[14] Genetic variability is also dependent on position within the biofilm, and different genes for the same species are upregulated at specific depth locations shown by confocal laser scanning microscopy.[24] Specific species also produce certain proteins that help the biofilm shield itself from the environment. For example, *Pseudomonas aeruginosa* produces acyl-homoserine (AHL) as well as other rhamnolipids and polysaccharides that are important for adhesion, binding, and matrix formation.[14,25,26] *P aeruginosa* biofilms also upregulate a housekeeping catalase gene that renders it impenetrable to hydrogen peroxide solutions.[27] Certain protein upregulation has been found to be specific to each stage of biofilm development. Proteins related to metabolic pathways, transport, lipid biosynthesis reactions, adaptation, and protection are upregulated following adhesion. Overall, more than 800 different proteins are upregulated in the development of a *P aeruginosa* biofilm.[15]

Virulence

The presence of the biofilm itself causes a mechanical impedance of host healing mechanisms such as contraction and epithelization; however, it also causes a dysregulation of inflammatory proteins by affecting intracellular signaling.[9] Keratinocyte migration is inhibited by surface receptors that sense the glycocalyx and bacterial products, and halt migration.[28] The early formation around blood vessels seen in the attachment phase may be important in bacterial invasion of vasculature and systemic spread.[11] In addition, the variability of the detachment process in the biofilm's life cycle also contributes to its virulence. Small clusters and cell groups are shed more frequently in planktonic form, but larger areas containing high amounts of biomass comprise 60% of total shed area, which may allow for the critical mass necessary to promote infection or attachment to a different host.[19]

CHARACTERIZATION OF BIOFILMS

In the clinical setting, specimen culture is the gold standard for microbial characterization. As the structure of the biofilm has been studied, it has become increasingly clear that cultures are an ineffective method for characterization of biofilm ecology. A few specific biofilm properties contribute to this conclusion. First, standard clinical cultures are inherently biased toward planktonic organisms that grow well in laboratory media, and thereby results may reflect the growth of organisms that only play a small role in the overall pathogenesis of a wound.[29,30] In addition, because of the alginate matrix in which they are bound, specimens require processing to break the carbohydrate bonds and release the encased microbes. One reported innovative approach was the use of sonication on infected bioprosthesis samples in the setting of preoperative antibiotic usage in knee and hip prosthesis surgery. The cultured results after using this technique were significantly more sensitive than standard culture techniques.[31] However, these methods have not been standardized in clinical practice and are prone to technical error. Given these limitations, other methods of direct visualization and molecular techniques have been used to study the structure and behavior of biofilms.[21,32]

Direct Observations

Microscopy has been used extensively in biofilm research, including light, electron, epifluorescence, and transmission microscopy techniques. The clinical findings on microscopy suggestive of the presence of biofilm are dense bacterial clusters in the presence of extracellular polymeric substances.[4] Microscopic examination demonstrates the interconnected fibrous network of extracellular polymeric substances at varied thickness, activities, species and species viability of microcolonies, and the cross-linking of bacterial cells within EPS.[6,12,15,33] Peptide nucleic acid (PNA) evaluation using fluorescence in situ hybridization (FISH) is another modality useful in visualizing the overall bioburden in the microcolonies that may not be appreciated by specimen culture.[10,20,21,24] These modalities have also been used to evaluate the efficacy of proposed antibiofilm compounds.[5]

Molecular Techniques

There are several molecular techniques used to evaluate biofilms in the research setting. The 3 main molecular techniques currently used are based on the polymerase chain reaction (PCR). The use of PCR first requires nucleic acid extraction from the sample. Validated methods of nucleic acid extraction from biofilms include boiling, phenolic chaotropic reagents, silica gel, and chemical extraction. Early in the history of wound biofilm research, commercial kits available for other substances such as soil, food, and sputum were used.[4,5,30,32,34–37] Use of the standard PCR in molecular diagnostics for biofilm is limited for various reasons. First, specific primer sets are used, limiting the result in a polymicrobial specimen, and the amplified result is confounded in the setting of mixed genetic material. In addition, the standard method is unable to evaluate quantitatively the genetic copies within a sample.

This problem of quantitative analysis was solved by the use of real-time or quantitative PCR, which reads the amplification during the reaction and therefore can tell how many genetic copies are being amplified. The use of quantitative PCR can quantify each species contribution to the overall bioburden of a biofilm and determine markers that identify resistance to specific antibiotic classes. A cost analysis of this technique has shown equivalence with culture-based analysis. Use of this technology in several studies has supported the theory that many biofilm pathogens are viable but not routinely culturable.[5,29,37,38]

The difficulty of PCR to meaningfully amplify a polymicrobial sample has been solved with the use of broad primer–based PCR or multiplex PCR. Multiplex PCR consists of multiple primers based on the genetically conserved segment of DNA within species to produce amplicons of varying sizes that are specific to different DNA sequences present; this is based on highly conserved regions in ribosomal RNA, signal recognition particles, and essential protein-encoding genes. By targeting conserved regions, variation within an amplified region is analyzed simultaneously, which is especially useful for mixed samples.[35,39] One commercial platform that uses this technique has been able to create an automated analysis of more than 1500 PCR reactions per day.[40] The limitation of broad-based PCR, however, is that it is zero sum in that the upper limit value is divided between the targets amplified.[35]

The use of molecular analysis on wounds has some inherent concerns. Some critics of this technique have been concerned that by evaluating the nucleic acid content of a biofilm, nonviable genetic material will be captured; this is more of a concern for DNA than RNA, as RNA has a very short half-life.[41] Past use of certain commercial kits for environmental pathogens, such as ones using ethidium monoazide bromide for muting nonviable DNA amplification, has been effective in soil samples but not in mammalian biofilm models.[41–43] PCR-based studies in middle ear effusions showed no detectable DNA after 1 to 3 days for heat-killed or purified DNA, whereas live bacteria persisted for several weeks even in those colonies with a culture-negative result.[44,45] The mixed results for determining the PCR capability of detecting nonviable genetic material may have to do with the wound itself. One possibility could be that wound mediators such as macrophages expedite the breakdown of purine and pyrimidine components of nonviable nucleic acid in a different way than could be observed in the studies on soil or food pathogens. For example, early work on purine release from wounded skeletal muscle shows rapid purine metabolism and suggests that a high-energy phosphate-promoting factor released by macrophages can affect the total nucleic acid present in a wound bed.[46]

After the genetic material is amplified, the genetic copies can be analyzed using various techniques. The main tests studied for use in biofilm thus far have been denaturing gradient gel electrophoresis (DGGE), pyrosequencing, and mass spectrometry. Some of the more sophisticated uses of DGGE have included a multistep nesting technique to help in uncoding complex polymicrobial samples.[4,30,32,34,47,48] Also, the use of rpo-B, which is a subunit of RNA polymerase, has been helpful in that it results in a single band on DGGE gel and can distinguish different species.[49] Pyrosequencing is the process of using single DNA strands to synthesize the complementary strand using DNA polymerase. This technique also has demonstrated extensive biodiversity in biofilm as compared with culture methods and different clusters of genomes related to distinct types of wounds.[32,36] A variant of pyrosequencing is called 16S 454 deep sequencing. This technique first fixes DNA fragments to beads, then uses PCR for amplification, followed by enzymatic sequencing using DNA polymerase and other enzymes. This test is extremely sensitive and can evaluate 400 to 600 million base pairs per run; however, it is also very costly in terms of labor and time outside the confines of even a well-resourced research laboratory.[32,36] The Sanger method of sequencing, well known for its usefulness on the human genome project, uses fluorescent labeling of the nucleotides, creating a collection of DNA fragments that can be amplified and separated and ordered by capillary array electrophoresis (CAE).[32] Mass spectrometry uses the physical number of base pairs present to create spectral signals that can determine the base composition of each amplicon. The resultant ability to detect small differences in the composition of small quantities of nucleic acid has the potential to become the method of choice for high-output, accurate measure of DNA load in the clinical setting.[39,40,50–52] This tool has been a useful one for tracking epidemics and bioterrorism by identifying subtypes of all pathogens and emergence of new species, as well as viral loads after vaccines.[53–56]

BIOFILM ERADICATION

There are many methods and agents in use for treatment of wound biofilms. In general, these can be separated into the two categories of mechanical debridement and chemical debridement.

Mechanical Debridement

There are several tools useful for eradicating the biofilm. Some are more appropriately used in the operating room and others are better suited to the outpatient setting. The goal of mechanical debridement is to completely remove all necrotic tissue and biofilm in the wound bed while leaving viable tissue untouched. Some centers find it useful to paint a wound with methylene blue to determine depth and boundaries of the wound when there is contour present. This coloring allows easy identification of the wound bed and remaining biofilm surface during operative debridement. The basic premise of mechanical debridement is to alter wound anatomy by unroofing all undermining and sinus tracts, then removing all devitalized tissue including bone and slough.[7] For more extensive information on this topic please refer to the article by Michael Caldwell elsewhere in this issue.

Commercial tools for debridement

There are several commercial products in use for mechanical debridement. These tools have been anecdotally useful, but there is a paucity of clinical trials to support their efficacy over standard sharp surgical debridement. This area of research needs further pursuit, especially in the setting of biofilms. One of the most widely used methods is hydrosurgery, a unique technique in that it is tissue selective but provides thorough debridement of the wound bed by both cutting and aspirating the necrotic soft tissue. Hydrosurgery has been shown to be useful in the burn setting to debride contoured wounds, and in wound bed preparation before immediate split-thickness skin grafting in contaminated wounds.[57–59] Pulsed electric and radiofrequency stimulation has also shown benefit, with faster healing rates compared with controls.[60,61] Pressure irrigation and ultrasound have not been shown to be effective in debridement as of yet, and require further study.[62]

Wound dressings

The purpose of wound dressings is to help control the moisture in the wound bed and protect the granulating tissue from external or mechanical forces that would halt the healing process. The standard wet to dry dressing method used often in wound care is a form of mechanical debridement. There are many types of dressings available, and it is beyond the scope of this article to evaluate each. An exudative wound needs a dressing that will wick away the moisture, whereas a dry wound needs a dressing that will retain moisture and minimize desiccation. Negative pressure wound therapy is one very popular wound dressing in use that has shown great promise in its ability to control the moisture in exudative areas while also aiding the contractile forces and lessening the time to total closure. This therapy has been evaluated in clinical trials, but a recent meta-analysis found that many of the studies on negative pressure therapy are poorly executed or inconclusive.[63–65] There is a large body of anecdotal uses for negative pressure therapy that has significantly improved patient care in wound healing. The use of this therapy in the setting of biofilm, however, must be performed with caution. It is imperative to ensure that the wound bed is absent of any contamination before applying the negative pressure dressing as the dressing stays in place for several days. Another unique but effective wound dressing is the sterile larva of the species *Lucilia sericata*. These larvae provide specific debridement in only removing cell debris and nonviable tissue, and inhibiting proinflammatory responses of phagocytes while promoting tissue remodeling. Their major activity appears to be related to their excretions and secretions. Clinical trials have shown varied kill time and clinical effect, depending on the species of bacteria.[66]

Chemical Debridement

Several studies have confirmed that most of the commercial antimicrobial and topical enzymatic agents used in wound care are ineffective in biofilm penetration, and therefore fail to appropriately eliminate critical wound bacterial colonization and stimulate wound healing.[5,8,67,68] Agents such as bleach, silver-containing compounds, and antibiotics require up to 1000-fold higher solution concentrations to provide bactericidal effects within a biofilm as compared with their efficacy against planktonic bacterial forms.[5,68,69]

Autolytic

Autolytic dressings are designed to help the body use its own immunologic agents to eradicate wound debris. These dressings include agents that keep the wound bed moist and the exudate contained, so that the natural process of phagocytosis and debridement will occur. These agents include hydrogel, hydrocolloid, or transparent semiocclusive dressings. The debridement that occurs is selective only for the necrotic tissue and is highly dependent on a patient's overall health and innate healing ability.

Enzymatic

Chemical agents can be used to aid the body's ability to digest necrotic tissue. Certain agents are selective just for necrosis while others are not, and have the potential to endanger the granulation process and epithelization once the eschar is eliminated.

Antimicrobial

There are many antimicrobial agents used in wound care, either as topical agents or as impregnated dressings. These agents have had mixed results when tested for biofilm penetration and when used prophylactically to prevent biofilm formation after debridement. Ionic silver's effect in wound care is due to its interference with the electron transport system of bacteria and the disruption of the cytoplasmic membranes. When used against biofilms, it has required concentrations 10- to 100-times stronger than is needed for planktonic organisms. However, silver sulfasalizine dressings with stronger concentrations (5–10 µg/mL) have positive effects of 90% eradication within 24 hours and 100% eradication in 48 hours against microcolonies within a biofilm.[68,70] Iodine is another common agent used that has bactericidal and bacteriostatic properties against methicillin-resistant *Staphylococcus aureus* (MRSA) and other pathogens. A few trials in the setting of biofilm have shown that the cadexomer iodine form is effective for biofilm suppression, while not causing tissue damage to the wound bed.[71,72] Chlorine and bleach are other common agents in wound dressings; however, it appears that effective concentrations for bleach are 50-fold greater for biofilm, and chlorine does not reach greater than 20% of the bulk of the biofilm measured by a depth electrode.[5,73] Chlorhexidine and polyhexamide work by binding to the stratum corneum, thereby disrupting the microbial membranes. Their efficacy in the setting of biofilm is unclear.[71] Triclosan and gallium were shown to be inhibitory to the formation of biofilm.[5] Leptospermum honey, a common wound dressing in resource-poor areas, is biocidal, and up to 60 bacterial species are reportedly susceptible in either planktonic or biofilm form, including antibiotic-resistant strains such as MRSA. The active agents in honey are methylglyoxal (inhibits cell division), hydrogen peroxide, fructose (blocks bacterial binding), flavinoids, acids, and minerals.[74]

Antibiotics

The use of antibiotics in wounds is controversial. The historical practice of systemic antibiotics for chronic wounds is not well supported unless there is objective evidence of local and systemic infection. If the wound is brightly erythematous with induration and pain, and the patient has documented bacteremia, then the use of systemic antibiotics may be warranted. In wound biofilms without evidence of local infection or systemic spread, systemic antibiotic therapy has been shown to be marginally helpful, with as low as 25% to 30% efficacy.[8] By contrast, there has been widespread use of topical antibiotics in biofilms and chronic wounds. Evaluation of this practice has yielded mixed results. In large part, topical antibiotic solutions have been shown to be very effective in treating planktonic organisms, but without debridement or the use of detergent to dissolve the biofilm these agents are ineffective. Bacteria within biofilms are 1000 times more resistant to topical antibiotics than planktonic culture.[6,69] Biofilm resistance to topical antibiotics can be explained on 3 levels.[12] First, the glycocalyx prevents perfusion of biocides to the bacteria on the mechanical level, especially the alginate.[33] Second, the bacteria within a biofilm are often in a senescent state, making certain specific antibiotic actions obsolete. Third, if the antibiotics are able to penetrate the biofilm, their molecular structure might be altered by the pH within the biofilm and change the bioavailability of the agents.[13] Another difficulty in the use of topical antibiotics for biofilm is determining sensitivity. Standard cultures evaluating planktonic organisms are not useful in determining sensitivity of bacteria encased within the biofilm. One innovative solution suggested is the use of poloxamer gel as an in vitro model for culturing biofilm specimens and testing for antibiotic susceptibility.[75]

Detachment-Promoting Agents

The study of biofilm eradication has also focused on the detachment-promoting agents, which work on the EPS to dissolve the basic biofilm structure. Efficacy of these agents could allow for outpatient topical treatment of wound biofilms. These agents are primarily enzymatic and function to disrupt the carbohydrate structure. A few of the most commonly used agents are cellulose, polysaccharide depolymerase, alginate, lyase disaggregatase esterase, dispersin B, DNAase, and urea.[8,76] Some interesting new findings show that D-amino acids may play a role in spontaneous biofilm disassembly by causing the release of the linking amyloid fibers in the matrix, and show promise in acting as deterrents to biofilm formation when used prophylactically.[77]

Antibiofilm Agents

In some centers, specific antibiofilm agents have been used to decrease biofilm growth after debridement by interfering with the physiologic mechanism of the bacteria. Lactoferrin blocks bacterial surface attachment through its affinity for iron in an acidic environment. This affinity allows for bactericidal action by neutrophils and disruption of the matrix, due to increased membrane permeability from the release of lipopolysaccharides. This agent has also been shown to act synergistically with xylitol.[7,8,33] Xylitol impairs matrix development by inhibiting glycocalyces, and disrupts cell wall growth in gram-positive organisms.[7,8,33]

Ethylenediaminetetraacetic acid also limits attachment by decreasing iron availability, and has been included in topical wound gels to prevent biofilm formation.[7,8,13] Gallium has a similar ionic radius to iron and therefore can disrupt iron-dependent systems within bacteria.[5,7,8] Other agents that have been shown to be useful in biofilm inhibition are acetylsalicylic acid, RNA III inhibitory peptide, furanone, farnesol, and selenium.[8,78]

SUMMARY

- Biofilms are ubiquitous, and most chronic and some acute wounds will have a biofilm present.
- Biofilms are difficult to evaluate diagnostically in the clinical setting, and standard culture methods are inadequate for capturing the true bioburden present in the biofilm.

- New molecular techniques used in the research setting may be transferable to clinical practice, and provide the means for rapid detection and evaluation of biofilms in the future.
- Many commercial topical agents and wound dressings in use are ineffective against the biofilm matrix.
- Mechanical debridement is essential to eradicate the biofilm.
- Topical antimicrobial agents and antibiotics may be effective in the treatment of the wound bed after debridement in the prevention of biofilm reformation.

ACKNOWLEDGMENTS

The authors would like to thank Marie Fleisner from the Office of Scientific Writing and Publication at Marshfield Clinic Research Foundation, and Mary O'Toole from the Allegheny Center for Genomic Sciences, for management and editorial assistance in the preparation of this article.

REFERENCES

1. Costerton JW. Overview of microbial biofilms. J Ind Microbiol 1995;15(3):137–40.
2. Donlan RM, Costerton JW. Biofilms: survival mechanisms of clinically relevant microorganisms. Clin Microbiol Rev 2002;15(2):167–93.
3. Costerton JW, Montanaro L, Arciola CR. Biofilm in implant infections: its production and regulation. Int J Artif Organs 2005;28(11):1062–8.
4. James GA, Swogger E, Wolcott R, et al. Biofilms in chronic wounds. Wound Repair Regen 2008;16(1):37–44.
5. Sun Y, Dowd SE, Smith E, et al. In vitro multispecies Lubbock chronic wound biofilm model. Wound Repair Regen 2008;16(6):805–13.
6. Davis SC, Ricotti C, Cazzaniga A, et al. Microscopic and physiologic evidence for biofilm-associated wound colonization in vivo. Wound Repair Regen 2008;16(1):23–9.
7. Wolcott RD, Rhoads DD. A study of biofilm-based wound management in subjects with critical limb ischaemia. J Wound Care 2008;17(4):145–8, 150–2, 154–5.
8. Rhoads DD, Wolcott RD, Percival SL. Biofilms in wounds: management strategies. J Wound Care 2008;17(11):502–8.
9. Wolcott RD, Rhoads DD, Dowd SE. Biofilms and chronic wound inflammation. J Wound Care 2008;17(8):333–41.
10. Bjarnsholt T, Kirketerp-Møller K, Jensen PØ, et al. Why chronic wounds will not heal: a novel hypothesis. Wound Repair Regen 2008;16(1):2–10.
11. Schaber JA, Triffo WJ, Suh SJ, et al. *Pseudomonas aeruginosa* forms biofilms in acute infection independent of cell-to-cell signaling. Infect Immun 2007;75(8):3715–21.
12. Harrison-Balestra C, Cazzaniga AL, Davis SC, et al. A wound-isolated *Pseudomonas aeruginosa* grows a biofilm in vitro within 10 hours and is visualized by light microscopy. Dermatol Surg 2003;29(6):631–5.
13. Dunne WM Jr. Bacterial adhesion: seen any good biofilms lately? Clin Microbiol Rev 2002;15(2):155–66.
14. Hentzer M, Eberl L, Nielsen J, et al. Quorum sensing: a novel target for the treatment of biofilm infections. BioDrugs 2003;17(4):241–50.
15. Sauer K, Camper AK, Ehrlich GD, et al. *Pseudomonas aeruginosa* displays multiple phenotypes during development as a biofilm. J Bacteriol 2002;184(4):1140–54.

16. O'Toole GA, Kolter R. Flagellar and twitching motility are necessary for *Pseudomonas aeruginosa* biofilm development. Mol Microbiol 1998;30(2):295–304.
17. Purevdorj-Gage B, Costerton WJ, Stoodley P. Phenotypic differentiation and seeding dispersal in nonmucoid and mucoid *Pseudomonas aeruginosa* biofilms. Microbiology 2005;151(Pt 5):1569–76.
18. Costerton JW, Cheng KJ, Geesey GG, et al. Bacterial biofilms in nature and disease. Annu Rev Microbiol 1987;41:435–64.
19. Stoodley P, Wilson S, Hall-Stoodley L, et al. Growth and detachment of cell clusters from mature mixed-species biofilms. Appl Environ Microbiol 2001;67(12): 5608–13.
20. Fazli M, Bjarnsholt T, Kirketerp-Møller K, et al. Nonrandom distribution of pseudomonas aeruginosa and staphylococcus aureus in chronic wounds. J Clin Microbiol 2009;47(12):4084–9.
21. Kirketerp-Møller K, Jensen PØ, Fazli M, et al. Distribution, organization, and ecology of bacteria in chronic wounds. J Clin Microbiol 2008;46(8):2717–22.
22. Rasmussen K, Lewandowski Z. Microelectrode measurements of local mass transport rates in heterogeneous biofilms. Biotechnol Bioeng 1998;59(3):302–9.
23. Vadyvaloo V, Otto M. Molecular genetics of *Staphylococcus epidermidis* biofilms on indwelling medical devices. Int J Artif Organs 2005;28(11):1069–78.
24. Shemesh M, Tam A, Kott-Gutkowski M, et al. DNA-microarrays identification of *Streptococcus mutans* genes associated with biofilm thickness. BMC Microbiol 2008;8:236.
25. Manos J, Arthur J, Rose B, et al. Transcriptome analyses and biofilm-forming characteristics of a clonal *Pseudomonas aeruginosa* from the cystic fibrosis lung. J Med Microbiol 2008;57(Pt 12):1454–65.
26. Musk DJ Jr, Hergenrother PJ. Chemical countermeasures for the control of bacterial biofilms: effective compounds and promising targets. Curr Med Chem 2006; 13(18):2163–77.
27. Stewart PS, Roe F, Rayner J, et al. Effect of catalase on hydrogen peroxide penetration into *Pseudomonas aeruginosa* biofilms. Appl Environ Microbiol 2000;66(2):836–8.
28. Loryman C, Mansbridge J. Inhibition of keratinocyte migration by lipopolysaccharide. Wound Repair Regen 2008;16(1):45–51.
29. Wolcott RD, Dowd SE. A rapid molecular method for characterising bacterial bioburden in chronic wounds. J Wound Care 2008;17(12):513–6.
30. Freeman K, Woods E, Welsby S, et al. Biofilm evidence and the microbial diversity of horse wounds. Can J Microbiol 2009;55(2):197–202.
31. Trampuz A, Piper KE, Jacobson MJ, et al. Sonication of removed hip and knee prostheses for diagnosis of infection. N Engl J Med 2007;357(7):654–63.
32. Dowd SE, Sun Y, Secor PR, et al. Survey of bacterial diversity in chronic wounds using pyrosequencing, DGGE, and full ribosome shotgun sequencing. BMC Microbiol 2008;8:43.
33. Ammons MC, Ward LS, Fisher ST, et al. In vitro susceptibility of established biofilms composed of a clinical wound isolate of *Pseudomonas aeruginosa* treated with lactoferrin and xylitol. Int J Antimicrob Agents 2009;33(3):230–6.
34. Gillan DC, Speksnijder AG, Zwart G, et al. Genetic diversity of the biofilm covering *Montacuta ferruginosa* (Mollusca, bivalvia) as evaluated by denaturing gradient gel electrophoresis analysis and cloning of PCR-amplified gene fragments coding for 16S rRNA. Appl Environ Microbiol 1998;64(9):3464–72.
35. Ecker DJ, Drader JJ, Gutierrez J, et al. The Ibis T5000 universal biosensor: an automated platform for pathogen identification and strain typing. JALA Charlottesv Va 2006;11(6):341–51.

36. Dowd SE, Wolcott RD, Sun Y, et al. Polymicrobial nature of chronic diabetic foot ulcer biofilm infections determined using bacterial tag encoded FLX amplicon pyrosequencing (bTEFAP). PLoS One 2008;3(10):e3326.

37. Cury JA, Seils J, Koo H. Isolation and purification of total RNA from *Streptococcus mutans* in suspension cultures and biofilms. Braz Oral Res 2008;22(3): 216–22.

38. Drago L, Lombardi A, Vecchi ED, et al. Real-time PCR assay for rapid detection of *Bacillus anthracis* spores in clinical samples. J Clin Microbiol 2002;40(11): 4399.

39. Budowle B, Eisenberg AJ, Gonzalez S, et al. Validation of mass spectrometry analysis of mitochondrial DNA. Forensic Sci Int Genet 2009;2(1):527–8.

40. Sampath R, Hall TA, Massire C, et al. Rapid identification of emerging infectious agents using PCR and electrospray ionization mass spectrometry. Ann N Y Acad Sci 2007;1102:109–20.

41. Yang S, Rothman RE. PCR-based diagnostics for infectious diseases: uses, limitations, and future applications in acute-care settings. Lancet Infect Dis 2004; 4(6):337–48.

42. Pisz JM, Lawrence JR, Schafer AN, et al. Differentiation of genes extracted from nonviable versus viable micro-organisms in environmental samples using ethidium monoazide bromide. J Microbiol Methods 2007;71(3):312–8.

43. Birch L, Dawson CE, Cornett JH, et al. A comparison of nucleic acid amplification techniques for the assessment of bacterial viability. Lett Appl Microbiol 2001; 33(4):296–301.

44. Post JC, Aul JJ, White GJ, et al. PCR-based detection of bacterial DNA after antimicrobial treatment is indicative of persistent, viable bacteria in the chinchilla model of otitis media. Am J Otolaryngol 1996;17(2):106–11.

45. Aul JJ, Anderson KW, Wadowsky RM, et al. Comparative evaluation of culture and PCR for the detection and determination of persistence of bacterial strains and DNAs in the *Chinchilla laniger* model of otitis media. Ann Otol Rhinol Laryngol 1998;107(6):508–13.

46. Morris AS, Shearer JD, Forster J, et al. The relationship of purine metabolism to the macrophage-mediated increase of high energy phosphates in skeletal muscle. J Surg Res 1986;41(4):339–46.

47. Schabereiter-Gurtner C, Saiz-Jimenez C, Piñar G, et al. Phylogenetic 16S rRNA analysis reveals the presence of complex and partly unknown bacterial communities in Tito Bustillo cave, Spain, and on its Palaeolithic paintings. Environ Microbiol 2002;4(7):392–400.

48. Mühling M, Woolven-Allen J, Murrell JC, et al. Improved group-specific PCR primers for denaturing gradient gel electrophoresis analysis of the genetic diversity of complex microbial communities. ISME J 2008;2(4): 379–92.

49. Dahllöf I, Baillie H, Kjelleberg S. rpoB-based microbial community analysis avoids limitations inherent in 16S rRNA gene intraspecies heterogeneity. Appl Environ Microbiol 2000;66(8):3376–80.

50. Ecker DJ, Sampath R, Massire C, et al. Ibis T5000: a universal biosensor approach for microbiology. Nat Rev Microbiol 2008;6(7):553–8.

51. Weile J, Knabbe C. Current applications and future trends of molecular diagnostics in clinical bacteriology. Anal Bioanal Chem 2009;394(3):731–42.

52. Muddiman DC, Anderson GA, Hofstadler SA, et al. Length and base composition of PCR-amplified nucleic acids using mass measurements from electrospray ionization mass spectrometry. Anal Chem 1997;69(8):1543–9.

53. Ecker DJ, Massire C, Blyn LB, et al. Molecular genotyping of microbes by multilocus PCR and mass spectrometry: a new tool for hospital infection control and public health surveillance. Methods Mol Biol 2009;551:71–87.

54. Sampath R, Russell KL, Massire C, et al. Global surveillance of emerging influenza virus genotypes by mass spectrometry. PLoS One 2007;2(5):e489.

55. Ecker DJ, Sampath R, Blyn LB, et al. Rapid identification and strain-typing of respiratory pathogens for epidemic surveillance. Proc Natl Acad Sci U S A 2005;102(22):8012–7.

56. Grant RJ, Baldwin CD, Nalca A, et al. Application of the Ibis-T5000 pan-Orthopoxvirus assay to quantitatively detect monkeypox viral loads in clinical specimens from macaques experimentally infected with aerosolized monkeypox virus. Am J Trop Med Hyg 2010;82(2):318–23.

57. Vanwijck R, Kaba L, Boland S, et al. Immediate skin grafting of sub-acute and chronic wounds debrided by hydrosurgery. J Plast Reconstr Aesthet Surg 2010;63(3):544–9.

58. Caputo WJ, Beggs DJ, DeFede JL, et al. A prospective randomised controlled clinical trial comparing hydrosurgery debridement with conventional surgical debridement in lower extremity ulcers. Int Wound J 2008;5(2):288–94.

59. Rappl T, Regauer S, Wiedner M, et al. [Clinical experiences using the Versajet system in burns: indications and applications]. Handchir Mikrochir Plast Chir 2007;39(5):308–13 [in German].

60. Feedar JA, Kloth LC, Gentzkow GD. Chronic dermal ulcer healing enhanced with monophasic pulsed electrical stimulation. Phys Ther 1991;71(9):639–49.

61. Porreca EG, Giordano-Jablon GM. Treatment of severe (Stage III and IV) chronic pressure ulcers using pulsed radio frequency energy in a quadriplegic patient. Eplasty 2008;8:e49.

62. Ramundo J, Gray M. Is ultrasonic mist therapy effective for debriding chronic wounds? J Wound Ostomy Continence Nurs 2008;35(6):579–83.

63. Venturi ML, Attinger CE, Mesbahi AN, et al. Mechanisms and clinical applications of the vacuum-assisted closure (VAC) device: a review. Am J Clin Dermatol 2005; 6(3):185–94.

64. Armstrong DG, Lavery LA, Boulton AJ. Negative pressure wound therapy via vacuum-assisted closure following partial foot amputation: what is the role of wound chronicity? Int Wound J 2007;4(1):79–86.

65. Gregor S, Maegele M, Sauerland S, et al. Negative pressure wound therapy: a vacuum of evidence? Arch Surg 2008;143(2):189–96.

66. van der Plas MJ, Jukema GN, Wai SW, et al. Maggot excretions/secretions are differentially effective against biofilms of *Staphylococcus aureus* and *Pseudomonas aeruginosa*. J Antimicrob Chemother 2008;61(1):117–22.

67. Bjarnsholt T, Kirketerp-Møller K, Kristiansen S, et al. Silver against *Pseudomonas aeruginosa* biofilms. APMIS 2007;115(8):921–8.

68. Ceri H, Olson ME, Stremick C, et al. The Calgary biofilm device: new technology for rapid determination of antibiotic susceptibilities of bacterial biofilms. J Clin Microbiol 1999;37(6):1771–6.

69. Percival SL, Bowler P, Woods EJ. Assessing the effect of an antimicrobial wound dressing on biofilms. Wound Repair Regen 2008;16(1):52–7.

70. White RJ, Cutting K, Kingsley A. Topical antimicrobials in the control of wound bioburden. Ostomy Wound Manage 2006;52(8):26–58.

71. Akiyama H, Oono T, Saito M, et al. Assessment of cadexomer iodine against *Staphylococcus aureus* biofilm in vivo and in vitro using confocal laser scanning microscopy. J Dermatol 2004;31(7):529–34.

72. De Beer D, Srinivasan R, Stewart PS. Direct measurement of chlorine penetration into biofilms during disinfection. Appl Environ Microbiol 1994;60(12):4339–44.

73. Merckoll P, Jonassen TØ, Vad ME, et al. Bacteria, biofilm and honey: a study of the effects of honey on "planktonic" and biofilm-embedded chronic wound bacteria. Scand J Infect Dis 2009;41(5):341–7.

74. Clutterbuck AL, Cochrane CA, Dolman J, et al. Evaluating antibiotics for use in medicine using a poloxamer biofilm model. Ann Clin Microbiol Antimicrob 2007;6:2.

75. Xavier JB, Picioreanu C, Rani SA, et al. Biofilm-control strategies based on enzymic disruption of the extracellular polymeric substance matrix—a modelling study. Microbiology 2005;151(Pt 12):3817–32.

76. Kolodkin-Gal I, Romero D, Cao S, et al. D-amino acids trigger biofilm disassembly. Science 2010;328(5978):627–9.

77. Tran PL, Hammond AA, Mosley T, et al. Organoselenium coating on cellulose inhibits the formation of biofilms by *Pseudomonas aeruginosa* and *Staphylococcus aureus*. Appl Environ Microbiol 2009;75(11):3586–92.

Unusual Causes of Cutaneous Ulceration

Jaymie Panuncialman, MD[a,b], Vincent Falanga, MD[a,b,c,d],*

KEYWORDS

- Inflammatory ulcers • Pyoderma gangrenosum • Vasculitis
- Calciphylaxis • Cryofibrinogenemia

Skin ulceration represents a difficult clinical problem and a major source of morbidity for patients. The patient's quality of life is also significantly affected by pain, swelling, and management of wound drainage. Localized infection, wound colonization, and systemic symptoms add to the morbidity and can lead to amputation and mortality. Wound care and therapy can be very challenging, and the use of wound dressings must be done on a rational basis and must not be too cumbersome or uncomfortable. Also, cutaneous ulcers take a considerable length of time to heal. The limitations to the patients' mobility, social interactions, and their ability to work result in feelings of helplessness and depression.[1] Most cutaneous ulcers of the lower extremity are caused by venous insufficiency, arterial insufficiency, or neuropathy (especially of diabetic cause), and in general such ulcers are not difficult to diagnose. However, ulcers associated with or caused by systemic inflammatory conditions are often a major diagnostic and therapeutic challenge. The authors generally call these chronic ulcerations inflammatory ulcers (ie, pyoderma gangrenosum [PG], vasculitic ulcers, cryoglobulinemic ulcers) because a major and primary component of their pathophysiology depends on inflammation and immunologic phenomena. However, this group of ulcers also includes conditions due to microcirculatory occlusion; a primary localized inflammatory component is less obvious in these conditions. Therefore, for the purpose of the authors' discussion in this article, they use a broad definition of inflammatory ulcers, which include these 2 aspects of chronic ulcers, which are not caused

---

The authors have no conflict of interest to declare.

This work was supported by the NIH Center of Biomedical Research Excellence (P20RR018757) at Roger Williams Medical Center (PI: F.V.).

[a] Department of Dermatology, Roger Williams Medical Center, 50 Maude Street, Providence, RI 02908, USA

[b] NIH Center of Biomedical Research Excellence, Roger Williams Medical Center, 50 Maude Street, Providence, RI 02908, USA

[c] Department of Dermatology, Boston University School of Medicine, Boston, MA, USA

[d] Department of Biochemistry, Boston University School of Medicine, Boston, MA, USA

* Corresponding author. Department of Dermatology, Roger Williams Medical Center, 50 Maude Street, Providence, RI 02908.

E-mail address: vfalanga@bu.edu

by classical vascular diseases or neuropathy. As with most complex conditions, inflammatory ulcers require a careful multidisciplinary consultation and treatment approach. The internist, dermatologist, surgeon, and rheumatologist are often called to contribute their expertise to establish the diagnosis and coordinate care.

BASIC APPROACH TO PATIENTS WITH INFLAMMATORY ULCERS

The diagnosis of inflammatory ulcers begins with a detailed history taking. Several important questions need to be to be asked (from the patient/records or elicited by physical examination). The following is a reasonable list: What was the primary lesion? How did the lesion progress? How fast was the progression to ulceration? Was the lesion painful? What management and treatment interventions took place and have they improved or worsened the condition? Has there been a similar problem in the past? Were any new medications started over the last couple of months? Was a surgical procedure performed in the last several months? Have there been any changes in the patient's general health? A thorough review of the systems provides clues to diagnosis. A past medical history of connective tissue diseases (CTDs), diabetes, heart disease, kidney disease, inflammatory bowel disease (IBD), hepatitis, hypertension, coagulopathies, prior pregnancy, and malignancies help support or suggest a particular cause and diagnosis.

Physical examination needs to be comprehensive. Physical examination and attention to details must not be focused on the ulcer alone. Rather, careful observation of the surrounding skin and attention to other areas of the integument, such as the oral mucosa and nails, are essential. Cutaneous findings, such as livedo reticularis (a netlike violaceous discoloration surrounding a central paler area), palpable purpura, petechiae, nail splinter hemorrhages, and/or oral ulcers support an inflammatory cause of the ulceration. Lipodermatosclerosis, commonly presenting as redness, induration, and hyperpigmentation of the skin in the lower extremity, supports a diagnosis of venous insufficiency. Examination of the peripheral vascular system and testing for the presence of neuropathy are performed to exclude arterial insufficiency, venous disease, and neuropathy as causes of the ulceration. Examination of the ulcer involves recognizing features that are characteristic of certain types of ulcers and identifying problems that one can treat. For example, areas of necrosis and the presence of an eschar suggest a thrombotic disorder. Violaceous undermined borders are suggestive of PG. A reddish yellow plaque surrounding the ulcer is characteristic of necrobiosis lipoidica diabeticorum (NLD), which is typically associated with diabetes. Ulcers are often complicated by swelling, infection, irritant contact dermatitis from the wound drainage or dressings, or an allergic contact dermatitis from topical medications and dressings. An ulcer with foul odor and purulent drainage is most likely secondarily infected or heavily colonized and benefits from systemic/topical antibiotics or topical antiseptic treatment. Areas with necrosis and eschar formation in a patient with good pulses benefit from surgical debridement, most importantly in diabetic patients. Leg swelling should be addressed with compression, when the compression does not compromise blood supply. Use of a scoring system in addition to ulcer size may be a good objective way to track improvement (**Fig. 1**). As always, the wound bed must be optimized according to the established principles of wound bed preparation to promote healing and to make available treatments more effective.[2] Pain management is important to ensure compliance with treatment; referral to a pain management service may sometimes be necessary. Therefore, as just discussed, the workup and approach to inflammatory ulcers still require careful attention to the principles of general wound care and management.

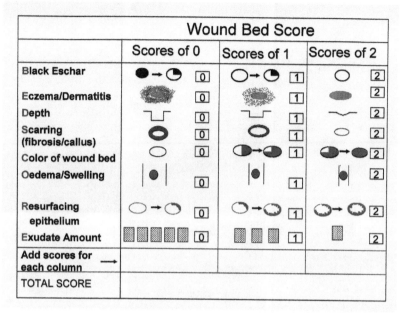

Fig. 1. Wound bed score (WBS) and its individual features. The total WBS adds each individual score for each characteristic to give a total score. ●, percentage of eschar present (>25, 1%–25%, none); ●, severity of periulcer dermatitis (severe, moderate, none, or mild); ⌣, depth of the wound (severely depressed or raised compared with periwound skin); ○, severity of callus/fibrosis (severe, moderate, none, or minimal); ●, percentage of pink granulation tissue present (<50%, 50%–75%, >75%); ●, severity of edema (severe, moderate, none, or mild); ○, percentage of healing edges (<25%, 25%–75%, >75%); ▨, frequency of dressing changes (severe, moderate, none, or mild). (*Courtesy of* Vincent Falanga, MD, Providence, RI. Copyright © 2009.)

Some of the main causes of inflammatory ulcers may be classified into the following primary or associated categories: immunologic conditions (ie, collagen vascular diseases and vasculitis), thrombotic or hypercoagulable states (ie, cholesterol embolization and the antiphospholipid syndrome), PG, and necrobiosis lipoidica (**Fig. 2**).

SPECIFIC INFLAMMATORY CONDITIONS
PG

PG was first described in patients with rapidly progressive, painful ulcers with violaceous undermined borders.[3] It is a disorder characterized by pathergy and the development of a larger ulcer on debridement or with trauma.[4] When already present, it can also develop in other, distant, seemingly unrelated areas of the skin; hence autologous grafting is a relative contraindication in these patients. Several clinical variants of PG have been recognized. The classic variant starts as a pustule that develops into a rapidly enlarging ulcer with undermined borders, surrounding erythema, and a purulent base. Among other systemic conditions, PG is associated with rheumatoid arthritis, IBD, Bechet disease, a monoclonal gammopathy (typically IgA), and myeloproliferative disease; many cases are idiopathic.[5] The pustular variant of PG manifests as painful pustules with an inflamed border and may not necessarily progress to frank ulceration. The skin manifestations of PG often parallel the severity of the underlying systemic disease and often resolve with control of their acute flare.[6] The bullous

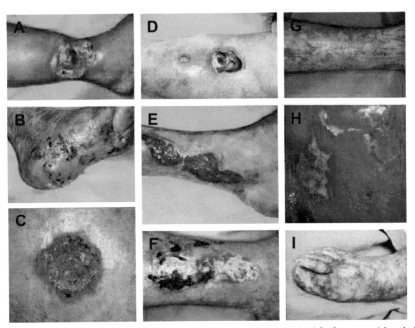

Fig. 2. Examples of some inflammatory ulcers. (*A*) PG in a patient with rheumatoid arthritis. (*B*) The more granulomatous appearance of PG. (*C*) Typical PG with purple edges. (*D*) Undermined ulcer of PG. (*E*) The undulating borders of a rheumatoid ulcer. (*F*) Eschar in an ulcer caused by polyarteritis nodosa. (*G*) Same ulcer shown in (*F*), after successful use of immunosuppressants. (*H*) The angular ulcers seen in patients with collagen vascular diseases, often mimicking factitial ulcers. (*I*) Livedo reticularis and small ulcers in a patient with cholesterol embolization. (*Courtesy of* Vincent Falanga, MD, Providence, RI. Copyright © 2002.)

variant of PG is characterized by the presence of painful bullae, which progress to superficial erosions and are associated with myeloproliferative disorders.[7] The vegetative variant is a superficial painless ulcer with undermined edges. This ulcer slowly enlarges and may be exophytic with no clear pattern of specific associated disease.[8] Parastomal PG presents as a nonhealing ulcer next to a colostomy site. This PG should be considered in all patients with IBD and a peristomal ulceration; the ulcer is typically quite refractory to local wound care approaches.[9,10] Extracutaneous involvement of PG has been reported as cavitary lung lesions, pulmonary infiltrates, episcleritis, development of a psoas muscle abscess, and splenic abscesses.[11–14]

The onset of the systemic condition may precede, follow, or occur simultaneously with PG; they may also run an independent course. Asymmetric seronegative monoarticular inflammation involving large joints is also associated with PG. A monoclonal IgA gammopathy can be present in the setting of PG and is usually benign, although the development of multiple myeloma has been reported.[5] Systemic malignancy has been estimated to occur in 7% of patients with PG, with leukemia being the most common neoplasm.[7] Certain drugs have also been implicated in the development of PG (granulocyte-macrophage colony-stimulating factor, interferons, and antipsychotic drugs).[15–18] The pathogenesis of PG is poorly understood. However, PG is postulated to be the result of neutrophil dysfunction, which may either consist of a defect in chemotaxis or may be caused by neutrophil hyper-reactivity. Also, the clonality of T cells has been detected in patients with PG in the absence of myeloproliferative disease, possibly indicating an excessive response to antigenic stimuli.[19,20]

Vascular and other types of ulcers may be misdiagnosed as PG. This misdiagnosis can be a serious clinical problem because treatment of PG with immunosuppressants may ultimately worsen ulcers caused or complicated by infection or malignancy. For example, ulcers caused by atypical mycobacteria and deep fungal infections may be misdiagnosed as PG. Initial (and temporary) improvements in an ulcer on immuno-suppressive treatment do not prove that it represents PG and should be analyzed with caution. Similarly, it is important to reevaluate the diagnosis of PG when the ulcers are recalcitrant to immunosuppressive therapy. Other inflammatory ulcers improve with immunosuppression, such as those associated with leukocytoclastic vasculitis, Wegener granulomatosis (WG), cutaneous polyarteritis nodosa (PAN), or antiphospholipid antibody syndrome.[4]

PG is a diagnosis of exclusion, a fact that is not generally appreciated by many clinicians. Critical diagnostic procedures, including biopsy, and other laboratory workup are used to exclude other causes of the ulceration, such as infections, malignancies, CTDs, or vaso-occlusive conditions. A skin biopsy is important to rule out other diagnoses more than to confirm a diagnosis of PG; the histologic examination is never truly diagnostic and still requires exclusion of an infectious cause. An adequate technique would be to perform an excisional biopsy down to the subcutaneous tissue, obtaining enough tissue for histologic examination and culture for bacteria, fungi, and mycobacteria. Laboratory tests should include an analysis of and detection of abnormalities in complete blood count (CBC), erythrocyte sedimentation rate, cytoplasmic antineutrophil cytoplasmic autoantibody (c-ANCA) and perinuclear ANCA (p-ANCA), basic metabolic panel, serum protein electrophoresis, coagulation panel, antiphospholipid antibody, cryoglobulins, cryofibrinogen, chest radiography, colonoscopy, as well as venous and arterial studies.[4,21] A patient with IBD may have minimal or no symptoms but still have abnormalities on colonoscopy.

Biopsy findings of PG are variable, depending on the area biopsied and stage of the ulcer. A biopsy specimen taken from the erythematous zone peripheral to the ulcer might show thrombosis and a lymphocytic infiltrate, which when present around blood vessels might qualify as a lymphocytic vasculitis; in general, the term lymphocytic vasculitis is somewhat controversial. The necrotic undermined border and the ulcer would typically show a dense mixed infiltrate and abscess formation. Concomitant leukocytoclastic vasculitis (with destruction of dermal blood vessel walls) is not uncommon but may be secondary to severe inflammation of the skin or even infection.[22]

No prospective randomized trials have been performed to determine the optimal treatment of PG, and only a few studies with case numbers of more than 15 patients have been published. High oral doses of systemic corticosteroids (>60 mg/day) and cyclosporine are the best-documented treatments and are often used as first line therapy. Both medications are useful for immediate control of the disease but are not suitable for long-term use because of their side effects. It has been reported that methylprednisolone, 0.5 to 1.0 mg/kg/d, and cyclosporine, 5 mg/kg/d, alone or in combination can be of benefit within 24 hours.[23–27] Methylprednisolone might be preferable to prednisone, especially because prednisone needs to be converted to methylprednisolone in the liver for optimal effects. Oral corticosteroids should be given to patients with PG for at least several weeks because short tapering courses of corticosteroids (eg, over a week) are ineffective.[24] Pulse therapy with intravenous (IV) corticosteroids can lead to rapid improvement (**Fig. 3**). Therapy with IV methylprednisolone (1 g/d) for 3 to 5 days is the typical regimen. The authors prefer a duration of 5 days. In the authors' opinion, methylprednisolone IV pulse therapy is most safely performed with the patient on telemetry because unpredictable electrolyte imbalances

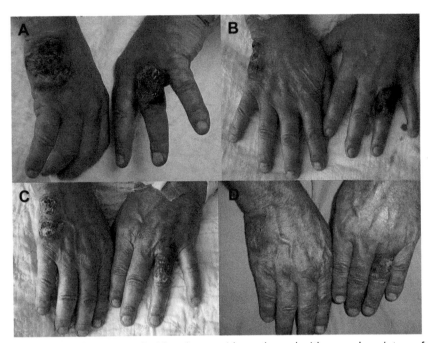

Fig. 3. Patient with PG treated with pulse steroids overlapped with mycophenolate mofetil as corticosteroid-sparing agent. (*A*) The appearance of a PG ulcer before treatment. (*B*) Dramatic improvement after the second day of pulse methylprednisolone. (*C*) Six days after pulse steroids the ulcers decreased markedly in size. (*D*) Healed ulcer 3 weeks after treatment. (*Courtesy of* Vincent Falanga, MD, Providence, RI. Copyright © 2007.)

may lead to fatal arrhythmias and even sudden death. Concomitant use of a diuretic is a relative contraindication to the use of pulse methylprednisolone therapy.[25,28,29]

Complications of therapy for PG need to be carefully considered. Patients on long-term systemic corticosteroids are at a risk of developing adrenal suppression, osteoporosis, peptic ulcers, and steroid psychosis, among other complications; avascular necrosis of the femoral head can occur very rapidly and at the onset of therapy. Nephrotoxicity, worsening of hypertension, congestive heart failure, and increased risk of malignancy are associated with cyclosporine. The authors prefer not to use cyclosporine in patients with hypertension or an evidence of coronary artery disease.

Tumor necrosis factor (TNF)-α antibodies or inhibitors have been used for the treatment of PG. The most studied anti–TNF-α drug for PG is infliximab. Infliximab is a humanized monoclonal antibody against TNF-α, which prevents the activation of proinflammatory cytokines resulting from the recruitment of inflammatory cells to tissue sites.[30,31] Generally, infliximab is administered with an induction dosing regimen infused as 5 mg/kg at weeks 0, 2, and 6. The optimal dosing of infliximab for PG is not known. There is controversy about whether infliximab is effective in patients with PG but without underlying IBD.[32–36] Immune-related side effects to infliximab, such as fever, chills, pruritus, urticaria, low or high blood pressure, and dyspnea, are most commonly reported. Infliximab therapy is associated with an increased risk of infections, including tuberculosis (TB). Reactivation of latent TB and hepatitis has been reported. It is not known whether infliximab increases the risk of solid tumors and malignancies; similar biologic drugs increase the risk of lymphoma. Infliximab treatment may not be suitable for patients with congestive heart failure. Rare cases of neurologic side effects, such as optic neuritis, demyelinating disorders, and multiple sclerosis, have been reported with infliximab. Furthermore, a lupuslike drug reaction has been associated with this biologic agent. Development of antibodies to infliximab increases the frequency of infusion reactions and shortens the duration of remission.[31]

Etanercept is a dimeric soluble form of the TNF-α receptor that prevents ligand binding to TNF receptors on the cell, thus rendering TNF-α inactive. Etanercept has been reported to be beneficial in the treatment of PG, at dosages of 25 to 50 mg weekly.[37–40] An advantage of using etanercept, over infliximab for example, is that it can be self-administered subcutaneously by the patient. Side effects of etanercept are similar to those observed with infliximab.

Other therapies for PG, such as mycophenolate mofetil, dapsone, thalidomide, and IV immunoglobulins, have been used alone or in combination with systemic corticosteroids.[41–45] For patients with limited and superficial PG, topical or intralesional corticosteroids and topical tacrolimus have been reported to be effective.[46,47] Goals of local wound care are to relieve pain, prevent colonization/infection, and support rapid reepithelialization. Bioengineered skin has been successfully used to stimulate reepithelialization and reduce pain while circumventing the problem of pathergy associated with the use of autologous grafts.[48]

Vasculitis

Inflammatory processes involving blood vessels can lead to skin ulceration. Vasculitis results from inflammation of the blood vessel wall, leading to hemorrhage, ischemia, and infarction. This sequence of events may be associated with CTDs (collagen vascular diseases), malignancy, or a drug reaction. Systemic symptoms of fevers, malaise, and joint pains necessitate further workup for a CTD.[49,50] Differently sized blood vessels may be affected. Vasculitis of the small dermal vessels manifests as palpable purpura, vesiculobullous lesions, and superficial ulcers with regular borders. Vasculitis of the muscular arteries presents as painful red nodules, punched-out irregularly shaped ulcers, or gangrene (**Fig. 4**).[51] Often, patients with vasculitis have systemic symptoms. The lower extremities are most commonly affected; involvement of the upper extremity, trunk, and head is an indication of more severe systemic disease.[52]

The key steps in the diagnosis of vasculitis are to determine the blood vessel damage and vessel size involved. The histologic patterns, supported by immunofluorescence findings, ANCA status, and workup for systemic disease, are the essential elements for diagnosis and for appropriate treatment.

Skin biopsies for routine studies as well as immunofluorescence should be performed on the most recent lesions, preferably those present for less than 48 hours. Because many ulcers due to vasculitis involve the medium-sized vessels, a skin biopsy extending to the subcutaneous fat is necessary. In skin lesions presenting with a livedoid pattern, the biopsy specimen must be taken from the paler center. Nonulcerated areas are preferred for biopsy. However, when biopsy specimens are taken from the ulcer bed, it is important to include the ulcer's edge (**Fig. 5**).[49,53,54] In addition to the biopsy, a CBC with differential, renal, and liver function tests; urinalysis; fecal occult blood testing; hepatitis B and C serologic tests; antiphospholipid antibody testing; immunoglobulin levels testing; complement levels testing; antinuclear antibody tests; rheumatoid factor testing; and p- and c-ANCA testing are recommended. Blood cultures and echocardiography may be considered in patients with a history of IV drug use or a high fever and a heart murmur.[51] Vasculitis may present as a single episode 7 to 10 days after exposure to a systemic drug or from infection; the vasculitis

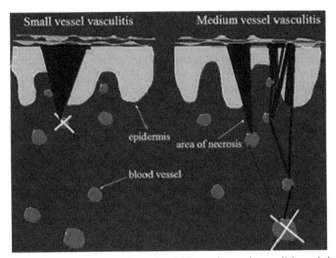

Fig. 4. Difference in small versus medium-sized (deeper) vessel vasculitis and the impact on skin findings. A superficial vasculitis (*left side*) leads to a wedge-shaped area of necrosis and thus, a well-defined and regular skin purpura or necrosis. Conversely, occlusion of a deep vessel (*right side*) leaves open the chance for anastomosing vessels to alter the effect at the skin. (*Courtesy of* Vincent Falanga, MD, Providence, RI. Copyright © 2007.)

may resolve in 1 to 3 months, but an intermittent and relapsing course with ulceration is seen in CTD-associated vasculitis, cryoglobulinemia, and malignancy.[49]

Microvascular occlusive processes owing to cryofibrinogenemia, the antiphospholipid antibody syndrome, hypercoagulable states from protein C and protein S deficiencies, or medication (such as warfarin) are important differential diagnoses to consider when livedoid skin lesions are observed. In many cases, the red or hyperpigmented cutaneous streaks are subtle (microlivedo) and do not resemble the full-blown netlike hyperpigmentation seen in livedo reticularis.

Leukocytoclastic vasculitis may present as superficial ulcerations and with hemorrhagic bullae on the lower portion of the leg and often without extracutaneous involvement. However, constitutional symptoms may be present. A minority of patients may have renal or gastrointestinal involvement. Skin biopsy observations show a small vessel vasculitis, whereas findings of immunofluorescence may reveal complement

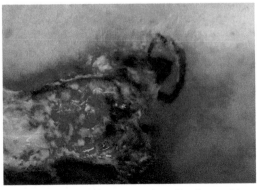

Fig. 5. Example of a biopsy for an inflammatory ulcer. Site for excisional biopsy marked on the edge of the ulcer including surrounding erythema.

and immunoglobulin deposition on vessel walls. Trigger factors for vasculitis are drugs, infection, and, rarely, an underlying CTD. Septic vasculitis is generally a small vessel vasculitis, as in leukocytoclastic vasculitis, that is immune-complex negative and is often caused by endocarditis and septicemia from a variety of microorganisms. Typical skin findings are purpura, pustules, hemorrhagic bullae, and ulcers. Blood cultures and echocardiography are essential for diagnosis.[55] Cutaneous small vessel vasculitis occurs frequently in systemic lupus erythematosus, rheumatoid arthritis, and Sjögren syndrome. In general, there is multiorgan involvement. The vasculitis may also affect larger blood vessels, as shown by the histologic examination. Physical findings vary from palpable purpura, to ulcers, and to digital gangrene, indicating significant arterial involvement.[51]

However, certain conditions affect larger blood vessels more commonly. WG is a disease that presents with lung, kidney, and skin involvement. It is associated with a destructive upper respiratory tract disease, saddle nose deformities, erosive sinusitis, and subglottic stenosis. Patients often have multiple lung nodules, infiltrates or alveolar hemorrhage, and segmental necrotizing glomerulonephritis. Skin findings may be palpable purpura, subcutaneous nodules, ulcers and digital infarcts, vesiculo-bullous lesions, and gingival hyperplasia. Vasculitis in this systemic condition affects small to medium-sized vessels. Biopsies of the upper respiratory tract may be diagnostic. A pattern of positive c-ANCA and PR-3 ANCA is strongly associated with WG. When untreated, the condition may approach a mortality of 80%.[51] Cutaneous PAN manifests as painful nodules progressing to ulceration with neuropathy. The clinical manifestations of PAN represent a spectrum, varying from nodules, livedo reticularis, and polyneuropathy to severe disease with cutaneous ulcers, pain, sensory neuropathy, fever, malaise, and arthralgia and progressive systemic disease; acral gangrene, foot drop, mononeuropathy multiplex, and musculoskeletal involvement can occur.[56] When the medium-sized blood vessel involvement of PAN is strongly suspected, multiple deep punch or incisional biopsies down to the fascia may be required to diagnose this disorder. Moreover, serial sections through the specimen are frequently necessary because the vasculitis is focal and segmental (**Fig. 6A**).[57]

In PAN, treatment of the underlying disease often leads to the resolution of the vasculitis. Mild disease may be treated with dapsone or colchicine. More severe or unresponsive PAN is managed with prednisone and/or with a corticosteroid-sparing agent. Systemic vasculitis with internal organ involvement may require the use of prednisone and cyclophosphamide, frequently in combination. Once remission has been achieved, maintenance with methotrexate or azathioprine alone is recommended.[58,59]

Cholesterol Embolism

Patients present with varied skin manifestations such as livedo reticularis, purpura, cyanosis, blue toes, digital gangrene, painful subcutaneous nodules, and renal failure; however, arterial hypertension is uncommon. Patients may also have fever, weight loss, myalgia, and anemia. Large vessels may be the source of the embolus, from which fragments separate and occlude the microcirculation. Several organ systems may be affected, with azotemia, abdominal pain from mucosal ulceration, gastrointestinal involvement from bleeding, ischemia, infarction, and perforation. Myocardial infarction, stroke, and transient ischemic attacks are not uncommon.[60-64] Cholesterol embolism (CE) occurs spontaneously or may be iatrogenic. Pathophysiologically, CE is the result of shearing forces causing atherosclerotic plaque rupture. Iatrogenic CE is caused by an endovascular surgical procedure or the initiation of anti-coagulant therapy (warfarin, heparin). However, in some cases, CE can develop weeks to months from the time of surgery or endovascular procedures or initiation of anticoagulation.[61,65]

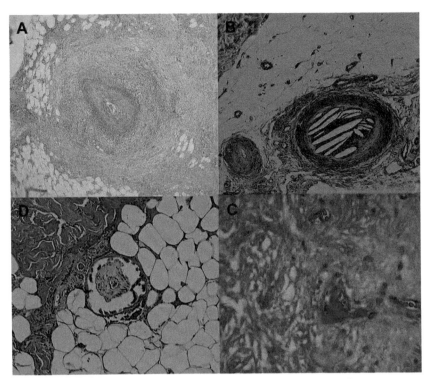

Fig. 6. Histologic findings in different inflammatory ulcers. (*A*) Dense inflammation around a medium-sized artery seen in polyarteritis nodosa. (*B*) Cleftlike spaces inside a vessel seen in cholesterol emboli. (*C*) Fibrin thrombi inside a vessel seen in cryofibrinogenemia. (*D*) Calcification of medial layer of a blood vessel seen in calciphylaxis. (*Courtesy of* Vincent Falanga, MD, Providence, RI. Copyright © 2010.)

Patients at high risk for CE are those with severe atherosclerotic disease. The formation of a fibrofatty plaque within the vessel wall, composed of a necrotic core of cell debris, foam cells, lipid and cholesterol crystals, and an overlying fibrous cap, is the central pathologic entity in atherosclerosis. When a plaque ruptures, a thrombus forms and breaks up, leading to less than 100 μm cholesterol fragments that embolize and occlude vessels in distant sites and affect different organ systems, including the skin. After the cholesterol crystals occlude the microcirculation, inflammation ensues, followed by a foreign body reaction with thrombus formation and eventual fibrosis. This sequence of events results in ischemia and infarction.[66] The presence of skin findings, such as livedo reticularis, microlivedo, or the blue toe syndrome, in addition to progressive renal failure is highly suggestive of cholesterol crystal embolization.[65] However, a skin biopsy specimen showing characteristic biconvex needlelike cleft in vessels on histologic examination is detected in up to 92% of patients and is specific for CE (see **Fig. 6**B, C).[61] An optimal site for the biopsy specimen is a tender nodule. However, the livedo area also has a high yield. CE has a high mortality rate; in one review of 221 patients mortality was 81%.[62]

An established treatment of CE is absent. When possible, anticoagulants should be withdrawn and further vascular procedures should be avoided after a diagnosis is established.[67,68] Aggressive supportive treatment has been reported to improve 1-year survival rates.[65] In this article, the approach included maintaining the patient's nutritional status, treating or preventing cardiac failure, and using hemodialysis. Systemic corticosteroids were started with evidence of recurrent CE or inflammation. However, the use of systemic corticosteroids is not consistently successful. Care must be exercised when patients are treated with corticosteroids because fluid retention and alterations in electrolyte imbalance further complicates the patient's cardiac status.[69] Statins, which can stabilize plaques, have been shown to decrease the risk of progression to end-stage renal disease and have improved the 1-year cumulative survival.[70] Surgical intervention (ie, removing the thrombus) in patients with CE is associated with significant morbidity, and its use is reserved for cases in which immediate survival is at stake.[65]

Calciphylaxis

Calciphylaxis has been classically described as the sudden development of tender, violaceous, and reticulate lesions that progress to necrotic ulcerations of the lower extremities in patients with renal failure on chronic hemodialysis. These ulcers heal poorly and are very painful. Areas commonly affected are those with thick adipose tissue, such as the abdomen, breasts, and buttocks. There is often an elevated parathyroid (PTH) level (secondary to renal failure), with abnormal calcium and phosphate metabolism.[71] Some investigators suggest that proximal ulcerations involving the abdomen and buttocks have a worse prognosis.[72] This classical concept and clinical context of calciphylaxis have been changing, as shown by several published case reports indicating a similar clinical course in the absence of renal failure, no obvious dysregulation of calcium and phosphate metabolism, and with normal PTH levels. However, a consistent histologic finding is calcification of the vessel walls, eventually leading to thrombosis and infarction of the skin. Other risk factors associated with the development of calciphylaxis include obesity, liver disease, systemic corticosteroid use, and an elevated calcium phosphorus product.[73] In addition, contributing factors are diabetes mellitus, warfarin use, decreased functional activities of protein C and protein S, vitamin D supplementation, and low albumin levels. Thus, in the proper clinical context, from physical examination and histologic findings, calciphylaxis should be considered even in the absence of kidney disease.[74] Peripheral pulses are preserved because only the smaller vessels are affected by calciphylaxis. Histologic findings of the cutaneous lesions show calcium deposits within the blood vessel walls, mainly in the media and intima of small arterioles and venules, frequently with a concentric, circumferential, and ringlike pattern (see **Fig. 6**D). These findings are seen in the dermis and the subcutaneous fat. Septal and lobular fat necrosis and epidermal ulceration with dermal necrosis are also identified.[75]

Treatment of calciphylaxis is mainly supportive. The goals of local wound care are to manage drainage with wound dressings, improve pain, treat infection, and stimulate healing (**Fig. 7**). If altered calcium metabolism and hyperparathyroidism are identified, treatment is directed to normalize these abnormalities. Several therapeutic measures have been tried with varied success. Simple approaches, such as establishing a diet with low phosphate intake and initiating oral phosphate binders, can be started. Bisphosphonates have been used because of their inhibitory effect on macrophages and proinflammatory cytokines to prevent further calcification. For example, pamidronate and etidronate have been used with some success.[76–78] Cinacalcet is a new calcimimetic agent that works by increasing the sensitivity of the calcium-sensing receptor on the PTH gland, thereby decreasing PTH levels and normalizing calcium levels.[79] This drug has been useful in patients with secondary hyperparathyroidism.[80,81] Sodium thiosulfate is thought to dissolve calcium deposits in tissues by forming soluble calcium thiosulfate complexes. The drug is given intravenously and has been reported to improve

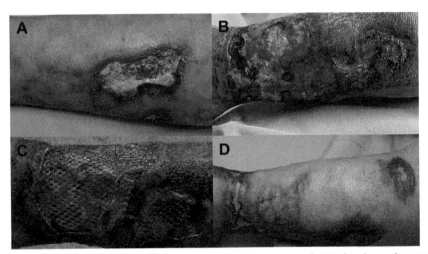

Fig. 7. Patient with calciphylaxis without renal failure, normal PTH levels, and normal calcium and phosphate product. (*A*) Painful ulcer with background livedo reticularis. (*B*) Worsening ulcer not responsive to pulse steroids, azathioprine, pentoxifylline, antibiotics, and debridement. Skin biopsy showed calciphylaxis. (*C*) Repeat debridement, IV antibiotics, and bioengineered skin applied to ulcer with good response; azathioprine discontinued after 1 month; compression therapy, pain management, and antiseptic dressings were used. (*D*) Ulcer healed after 3 months. (*Courtesy of* Vincent Falanga, MD, Providence, RI. Copyright © 2006.)

pain and wound healing.[82–84] In patients with calciphylaxis, parathyroidectomy and elevated PTH benefits wound healing and improves short-term mortality; the long-term benefits of this approach are unknown.[85–87]

The prognosis of calciphylaxis is generally poor, and the condition is associated with a mortality as high as 60% to 80%.[73] Sepsis occurs commonly, with ulceration as the probable portal of entry for infection.

Cryofibrinogenemia and Cryoglobulinemia

Signs and symptoms of cryofibrinogenemia are caused by cutaneous ischemia. Patients present with livedo reticularis or subtle areas of microlivedo, purpura, ecchymoses, and painful ulcerations that, strangely, are not commonly precipitated by cold ambient temperatures. Systemic symptoms of malaise and fever are common. Often, there is an underlying inflammatory disease, such as malignancy, diabetes mellitus, collagen vascular disease, or an infection. Essential cryofibrinogenemia occurs without a secondary cause and should be considered in healthy patients presenting with unexplained areas of cutaneous ischemia.[88] Rarely, other thrombotic events, such as myocardial infarction, thrombophlebitis, and cerebral infarction, are seen. Paradoxic spontaneous bleeding caused by consumption of clotting factors may occur.[88]

One needs to contrast cryofibrinogenemic versus cryoglobulinemic ulcers. The diagnosis of cryofibrinogenemic ulcers is made in a clinical setting of sudden onset of skin changes and ulcerations in the presence of elevated plasma cryofibrinogen and without serum cryoglobulins and evidence of other inflammatory causes of micro-occlusive diseases; the relationship of onset of pain, discomfort, and ulceration to cold exposure is uncommon. In contrast, cryoglobulinemic ulcers are definitely accompanied by purpura triggered by cold exposure or prolonged standing plus arthralgia and weakness; cryoglobulins are detected in serum. Cryoglobulins are associated with CTDs, hematologic malignancies, and hepatitis. Cryofibrinogenemia is commonly idiopathic but can be associated with myeloproliferative disorders and CTDs. Treatment of the underlying disease causing these cryoproteinemias leads to the improvement of symptoms and physical findings.

On biopsy of ulcers due to cryoproteinemias, small and medium-sized vessel vasculitis is seen. In terms of distinction, cryofibrinogens are a cold insoluble complex of fibrin, fibrinogen, and fibrin split products with albumin, plasma proteins, and immunoglobulins. Cryofibrinogen forms a clot with thrombin and reversibly precipitates in plasma at 4°C,[89] whereas cryoglobulins are cold-precipitating immunoglobulins in serum and dissolve when warmed. Skin biopsy findings showing fibrin occluding the dermal blood vessels, angiogram with abrupt occlusion of small to medium-sized arteries, and elevation of serum levels of α1-antitrypsin and α2-macroglobulin support a diagnosis of cryofibrinogenemia. High levels of α1-antitrypsin and α2-macroglobulin inhibit plasmin and fibrinolysis, which leads to the thrombotic occlusion of small to medium-sized arteries by the cryofibrinogens.[90,91] The detection of cryofibrinogens in plasma requires special handling and attention. Blood must be collected in tubes containing oxalate, citrate, or ethylenediaminetetraacetic acid as the anticoagulant. After collection, the blood must be quickly centrifuged at 37°C. Blood should also be collected in a plain glass tube, allowed to clot, and then processed in a similar fashion to detect the presence of cryoglobulins.

Treatment of cryofibrinogenemic ulcers includes avoidance of cold exposure and local wound care. The anabolic steroid stanozolol has an established fibrinolytic effect and has been used with considerable success in the past.[92,93] However, this drug has now been withdrawn from the market and is no longer easily available as a reliable preparation. However, the authors have used danazol with success (Vincent Falanga, unpublished data, 2010). Systemic corticosteroids alone do not appear to be an effective therapy. Treatment of the underlying condition may lead to improvement. Plasmapheresis has been effective in a few reports.[93–97] The authors have had success with the use of combined pentoxifylline and colchicine in one patient with cryofibrinogenemic ulcers (**Fig. 8**).[98]

NLD

NLD is characterized by single or multiple asymptomatic red to yellow shiny plaques that gradually enlarge and within which, because of atrophy, dermal blood vessels are readily apparent. Ulceration is a complication of NLD and commonly

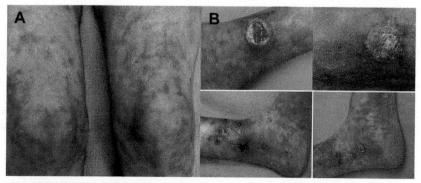

Fig. 8. Patient with cryofibrinogenemia. (*A*) Typical presentation of livedo reticularis. (*B*) Ulcers healed with compression pentoxifylline and colchicine. (*Courtesy of* Vincent Falanga, MD, Providence, RI. Copyright © 2005.)

develops after trauma to the lesions. Almost all patients with NLD have diabetes mellitus, or will develop it, or have a strong family history of it. However, less than 1% of diabetic patients have NLD.[99,100] The pathogenic steps leading to NLD are unknown. Biopsy of the lesions shows an atrophic epidermis and dermal areas of necrobiotic collagen surrounded by palisading histiocytes and extending to the subcutaneous fat. Spontaneous resolution of NLD has been reported to occur in about 20% of cases. A variety of treatments have been used for the treatment of NLD, including topical and intralesional corticosteroids, topical tacrolimus, psoralens plus ultraviolet A, and antimalarials. In patients with severe ulcerations with NLD, infliximab, etanercept, pentoxifylline, cyclosporine, and thalidomide have been used. Tight control of the patient's diabetes does not improve necrobiosis lipoidica.[101–108]

Warfarin-Induced Skin Necrosis

Sudden development of paresthesia, edema, petechiae, and ecchymoses progressing to full-thickness necrosis and deep ulcers within 3 to 10 days after the initiation of warfarin therapy should alert the clinician to the possibility of warfarin-induced skin necrosis (WISN).[109–111] WISN has been described in patients on anticoagulation, typically several days after therapy is stopped, or on re-treatment.[111–113] WISN is thought to be the result of a paradoxic hypercoagulable state, possibly because of the inhibition of vitamin K–dependent coagulation factors relative to other factors, thus producing a transient imbalance that predisposes to clotting. Deficiencies of protein C, protein S, and antithrombin III are considered a risk factor in the development of WISN. However, not all patients with protein C, protein S, and antithrombin III deficiencies develop WISN.[111,114–116]

The diagnosis of WISN is made by history taking and/or with a skin biopsy showing histologic findings of microthrombi and thrombi within the blood vessels of the dermis and subcutaneous tissue, including capillaries and venules; typically, there is no vasculitis. WISN needs to be differentiated from heparin-induced necrosis associated with heparin-induced thrombocytopenia and thrombosis (HITT) because both warfarin and heparin are frequently used concurrently. Both conditions present with skin necrosis. HITT is associated with a 50% reduction in platelet levels from baseline or a platelet count less than 150. However, platelet counts are frequently normal in HITT with skin ulceration. Symptoms begin at 4 to 12 days after starting heparin. The heparin PF-4 antibody is frequently present.[109,117] In contrast to WISN, the thrombus in HITT is mostly composed of platelets; true arterial thrombosis is common.[118]

Early diagnosis and immediate withdrawal of warfarin improves the prognosis of WISN. Replacement of clotting factors with fresh frozen plasma and the use of an alternate anticoagulant, such as heparin, may be required. Thus, it is important to distinguish between WISN and HITT because the mainstay of the treatment of HITT is discontinuation of heparin and switching to a different anticoagulant, such as argatroban; warfarin use alone is contraindicated in HITT.[119] Aggressive wound care and surgical intervention to remove the devitalized tissue are needed in many patients. Antibiotics are also frequently used but given with caution because antibiotics may alter or decrease the vitamin K–producing flora in the gut. Treatment with systemic corticosteroids or vasodilators has not improved WISN.[109,115] Useful measures to prevent warfarin necrosis are avoiding initial loading with warfarin and starting anticoagulation first with unfractionated heparin and overlapping with warfarin for about 5 days.[114,115]

SUMMARY

The sudden development of painful ulcerations with systemic symptoms in the context of an underlying disease, change in medications, and/or recent surgical intervention points to an inflammatory cause of the ulceration. A broad differential diagnosis exists for these ulcers. History taking, physical examination, and laboratory workup should be done, with careful consideration of an autoimmune, infectious, and/or occlusive process as the cause of ulceration. Providing wound care with the goals of optimizing wound healing by decreasing swelling, controlling the bacterial burden, and avoiding an irritant or allergic contact dermatitis are equally important. Treatment of the underlying illness often improves the ulceration as well. Because these diseases are not so common, no specific guidelines have been developed. Treatment should be carefully chosen, with emphasis on minimizing possible complications with its use. A multidisciplinary approach is necessary to manage these patients, and consultations with different specialties should be the rule. Re-evaluation of the diagnosis and management are advised if the ulcers fail to respond to treatment.

ACKNOWLEDGMENTS

This work was made possible by NIH Grant P20RR018757-07 (PI: Vincent Falanga) and by the grant's Imaging core and Regulatory and GMP core.

REFERENCES

1. Herber OR, Schnepp W, Rieger MA. A systematic review on the impact of leg ulceration on patients' quality of life. Health Qual Life Outcomes 2007;5:44.
2. Panuncialman J, Falanga V. The science of wound bed preparation. Clin Plast Surg 2007;34(4):621–32.
3. Brunsting LA, Goeckerman WH, O'Leary PA. Pyoderma (ecthyma) gangrenosum: clinical and experimental observations in 5 cases occurring in adults. Arch Derm Syphilol 1930;22:655–80.
4. Weenig RH, Davis MD, Dahl PR, et al. Skin ulcers misdiagnosed as pyoderma gangrenosum. N Engl J Med 2002;347(18):1412–8.
5. Powell FC, Schroeter AL, Su WP, et al. Pyoderma gangrenosum: a review of 86 patients. Q J Med 1985;55(217):173–86.
6. Powell FC, Su WP, Perry HO. Pyoderma gangrenosum: classification and management. J Am Acad Dermatol 1996;34(3):395–409 [quiz: 410–2].
7. Duguid CM, O'Loughlin S, Otridge B, et al. Paraneoplastic pyoderma gangrenosum. Australas J Dermatol 1993;34(1):17–22.
8. Langan SM, Powell FC. Vegetative pyoderma gangrenosum: a report of two new cases and a review of the literature. Int J Dermatol 2005;44(8):623–9.
9. Hughes AP, Jackson JM, Callen JP. Clinical features and treatment of peristomal pyoderma gangrenosum. JAMA 2000;284(12):1546–8.
10. Sheldon DG, Sawchuk LL, Kozarek RA, et al. Twenty cases of peristomal pyoderma gangrenosum: diagnostic implications and management. Arch Surg 2000;135(5):564–8 [discussion: 568–9].
11. Hubbard VG, Friedmann AC, Goldsmith P. Systemic pyoderma gangrenosum responding to infliximab and adalimumab. Br J Dermatol 2005;152(5):1059–61.
12. Field S, Powell FC, Young V, et al. Pyoderma gangrenosum manifesting as a cavitating lung lesion. Clin Exp Dermatol 2008;33(4):418–21.
13. Kanoh S, Kobayashi H, Sato K, et al. Tracheobronchial pulmonary disease associated with pyoderma gangrenosum. Mayo Clin Proc 2009;84(6):555–7.

14. Kruger S, Piroth W, Amo Takyi B, et al. Multiple aseptic pulmonary nodules with central necrosis in association with pyoderma gangrenosum. Chest 2001; 119(3):977–8.

15. Ross HJ, Moy LA, Kaplan R, et al. Bullous pyoderma gangrenosum after granulocyte colony-stimulating factor treatment. Cancer 1991;68(2):441–3.

16. Montoto S, Bosch F, Estrach T, et al. Pyoderma gangrenosum triggered by alpha2b-interferon in a patient with chronic granulocytic leukemia. Leuk Lymphoma 1998;30(1–2):199–202.

17. Sanders S, Busam K, Tahan SR, et al. Granulomatous and suppurative dermatitis at interferon alfa injection sites: report of 2 cases. J Am Acad Dermatol 2002;46(4):611–6.

18. Srebrnik A, Shachar E, Brenner S. Suspected induction of a pyoderma gangrenosum-like eruption due to sulpiride treatment. Cutis 2001;67(3):253–6.

19. Brooklyn TN, Williams AM, Dunnill MG, et al. T-cell receptor repertoire in pyoderma gangrenosum: evidence for clonal expansions and trafficking. Br J Dermatol 2007;157(5):960–6.

20. Magro CM, Kiani B, Li J, et al. Clonality in the setting of Sweet's syndrome and pyoderma gangrenosum is not limited to underlying myeloproliferative disease. J Cutan Pathol 2007;34(7):526–34.

21. Su WP, Davis MD, Weenig RH, et al. Pyoderma gangrenosum: clinicopathologic correlation and proposed diagnostic criteria. Int J Dermatol 2004;43(11): 790–800.

22. Su WP, Schroeter AL, Perry HO, et al. Histopathologic and immunopathologic study of pyoderma gangrenosum. J Cutan Pathol 1986;13(5):323–30.

23. Matis WL, Ellis CN, Griffiths CE, et al. Treatment of pyoderma gangrenosum with cyclosporine. Arch Dermatol 1992;128(8):1060–4.

24. Bennett ML, Jackson JM, Jorizzo JL, et al. Pyoderma gangrenosum. A comparison of typical and atypical forms with an emphasis on time to remission. Case review of 86 patients from 2 institutions. Medicine (Baltimore) 2000;79(1):37–46.

25. Chow RK, Ho VC. Treatment of pyoderma gangrenosum. J Am Acad Dermatol 1996;34(6):1047–60.

26. Vidal D, Puig L, Gilaberte M, et al. Review of 26 cases of classical pyoderma gangrenosum: clinical and therapeutic features. J Dermatolog Treat 2004; 15(3):146–52.

27. Elgart G, Stover P, Larson K, et al. Treatment of pyoderma gangrenosum with cyclosporine: results in seven patients. J Am Acad Dermatol 1991;24(1):83–6.

28. Prystowsky JH, Kahn SN, Lazarus GS. Present status of pyoderma gangrenosum. Review of 21 cases. Arch Dermatol 1989;125(1):57–64.

29. Johnson RB, Lazarus GS. Pulse therapy. Therapeutic efficacy in the treatment of pyoderma gangrenosum. Arch Dermatol 1982;118(2):76–84.

30. Reichrath J, Bens G, Bonowitz A, et al. Treatment recommendations for pyoderma gangrenosum: an evidence-based review of the literature based on more than 350 patients. J Am Acad Dermatol 2005;53(2):273–83.

31. Wolverton S. Comprehensive dermatologic drug therapy. 2nd edition. Philadelphia: Elsevier; 2007.

32. Adisen E, Oztas M, Gurer MA. Treatment of idiopathic pyoderma gangrenosum with infliximab: induction dosing regimen or on-demand therapy? Dermatology 2008;216(2):163–5.

33. Brooklyn TN, Dunnill MG, Shetty A, et al. Infliximab for the treatment of pyoderma gangrenosum: a randomised, double blind, placebo controlled trial. Gut 2006;55(4):505–9.

34. Regueiro M, Valentine J, Plevy S, et al. Infliximab for treatment of pyoderma gangrenosum associated with inflammatory bowel disease. Am J Gastroenterol 2003;98(8):1821–6.

35. Romero-Gomez M, Sanchez-Munoz D. Infliximab induces remission of pyoderma gangrenosum. Eur J Gastroenterol Hepatol 2002;14(8):907.

36. Mimouni D, Anhalt GJ, Kouba DJ, et al. Infliximab for peristomal pyoderma gangrenosum. Br J Dermatol 2003;148(4):813–6.

37. Roy DB, Conte ET, Cohen DJ. The treatment of pyoderma gangrenosum using etanercept. J Am Acad Dermatol 2006;54(3 Suppl 2):S128–34.

38. Goldenberg G, Jorizzo JL. Use of etanercept in treatment of pyoderma gangrenosum in a patient with autoimmune hepatitis. J Dermatolog Treat 2005;16(5–6): 347–9.

39. Pastor N, Betlloch I, Pascual JC, et al. Pyoderma gangrenosum treated with anti-TNF alpha therapy (etanercept). Clin Exp Dermatol 2006;31(1):152–3.

40. Charles CA, Leon A, Banta MR, et al. Etanercept for the treatment of refractory pyoderma gangrenosum: a brief series. Int J Dermatol 2007;46(10):1095–9.

41. Nousari HC, Lynch W, Anhalt GJ, et al. The effectiveness of mycophenolate mofetil in refractory pyoderma gangrenosum. Arch Dermatol 1998;134(12): 1509–11.

42. Daniels NH, Callen JP. Mycophenolate mofetil is an effective treatment for peristomal pyoderma gangrenosum. Arch Dermatol 2004;140(12):1427–9.

43. Hecker MS, Lebwohl MG. Recalcitrant pyoderma gangrenosum: treatment with thalidomide. J Am Acad Dermatol 1998;38(3):490–1.

44. Hagman JH, Carrozzo AM, Campione E, et al. The use of high-dose immunoglobulin in the treatment of pyoderma gangrenosum. J Dermatolog Treat 2001;12(1):19–22.

45. Altman J, Mopper C. Pyoderma gangrenosum treated with sulfone drugs. Minn Med 1966;49(1):22–6.

46. Lally A, Hollowood K, Bunker CB, et al. Penile pyoderma gangrenosum treated with topical tacrolimus. Arch Dermatol 2005;141(9):1175–6.

47. Kontos AP, Kerr HA, Fivenson DP, et al. An open-label study of topical tacrolimus ointment 0.1% under occlusion for the treatment of pyoderma gangrenosum. Int J Dermatol 2006;45(11):1383–5.

48. de Imus G, Golomb C, Wilkel C, et al. Accelerated healing of pyoderma gangrenosum treated with bioengineered skin and concomitant immunosuppression. J Am Acad Dermatol 2001;44(1):61–6.

49. Carlson JA, Cavaliere LF, Grant-Kels JM. Cutaneous vasculitis: diagnosis and management. Clin Dermatol 2006;24(5):414–29.

50. Carlson JA, Ng BT, Chen KR. Cutaneous vasculitis update: diagnostic criteria, classification, epidemiology, etiology, pathogenesis, evaluation and prognosis. Am J Dermatopathol 2005;27(6):504–28.

51. Chen KR, Carlson JA. Clinical approach to cutaneous vasculitis. Am J Clin Dermatol 2008;9(2):71–92.

52. Ioannidou DJ, Krasagakis K, Daphnis EK, et al. Cutaneous small vessel vasculitis: an entity with frequent renal involvement. Arch Dermatol 2002;138(3):412–4.

53. Grzeszkiewicz TM, Fiorentino DF. Update on cutaneous vasculitis. Semin Cutan Med Surg 2006;25(4):221–5.

54. Sais G, Vidaller A, Jucgla A, et al. Prognostic factors in leukocytoclastic vasculitis: a clinicopathologic study of 160 patients. Arch Dermatol 1998;134(3):309–15.

55. Carlson JA, Chen KR. Cutaneous vasculitis update: small vessel neutrophilic vasculitis syndromes. Am J Dermatopathol 2006;28(6):486–506.

56. Carlson JA, Chen KR. Cutaneous vasculitis update: neutrophilic muscular vessel and eosinophilic, granulomatous, and lymphocytic vasculitis syndromes. Am J Dermatopathol 2007;29(1):32–43.

57. Chen KR. Cutaneous polyarteritis nodosa: a clinical and histopathological study of 20 cases. J Dermatol 1989;16(6):429–42.

58. Lapraik C, Watts R, Scott DG. Modern management of primary systemic vasculitis. Clin Med 2007;7(1):43–7.

59. Bosch X, Guilabert A, Espinosa G, et al. Treatment of antineutrophil cytoplasmic antibody associated vasculitis: a systematic review. JAMA 2007;298(6):655–69.

60. Keon WJ, Heggtveit HA, Leduc J. Perioperative myocardial infarction caused by atheroembolism. J Thorac Cardiovasc Surg 1982;84(6):849–55.

61. Falanga V, Fine MJ, Kapoor WN. The cutaneous manifestations of cholesterol crystal embolization. Arch Dermatol 1986;122(10):1194–8.

62. Fine MJ, Kapoor W, Falanga V. Cholesterol crystal embolization: a review of 221 cases in the English literature. Angiology 1987;38(10):769–84.

63. Moolenaar W, Lamers CB. Cholesterol crystal embolisation to the alimentary tract. Gut 1996;38(2):196–200.

64. Rushovich AM. Perforation of the jejunum: a complication of atheromatous embolization. Am J Gastroenterol 1983;78(2):77–82.

65. Belenfant X, Meyrier A, Jacquot C. Supportive treatment improves survival in multivisceral cholesterol crystal embolism. Am J Kidney Dis 1999;33(5):840–50.

66. Gore I, McCombs HL, Lindquist RL. Observations on the fate of cholesterol emboli. J Atheroscler Res 1964;4:527–35.

67. Bruns FJ, Segel DP, Adler S. Control of cholesterol embolization by discontinuation of anticoagulant therapy. Am J Med Sci 1978;275(1):105–8.

68. Kawakami Y, Hirose K, Watanabe Y, et al. Management of multiple cholesterol embolization syndrome—a case report. Angiology 1990;41(3):248–52.

69. Donohue KG, Saap L, Falanga V. Cholesterol crystal embolization: an atherosclerotic disease with frequent and varied cutaneous manifestations. J Eur Acad Dermatol Venereol 2003;17(5):504–11.

70. Scolari F, Ravani P, Pola A, et al. Predictors of renal and patient outcomes in atheroembolic renal disease: a prospective study. J Am Soc Nephrol 2003;14(6):1584–90.

71. Dauden E, Onate MJ. Calciphylaxis. Dermatol Clin 2008;26(4):557–68, ix.

72. Oh DH, Eulau D, Tokugawa DA, et al. Five cases of calciphylaxis and a review of the literature. J Am Acad Dermatol 1999;40(6 Pt 1):979–87.

73. Weenig RH, Sewell LD, Davis MD, et al. Calciphylaxis: natural history, risk factor analysis, and outcome. J Am Acad Dermatol 2007;56(4):569–79.

74. Kalajian AH, Malhotra PS, Callen JP, et al. Calciphylaxis with normal renal and parathyroid function: not as rare as previously believed. Arch Dermatol 2009; 145(4):451–8.

75. Essary LR, Wick MR. Cutaneous calciphylaxis. An underrecognized clinicopathologic entity. Am J Clin Pathol 2000;113(2):280–7.

76. Monney P, Nguyen QV, Perroud H, et al. Rapid improvement of calciphylaxis after intravenous pamidronate therapy in a patient with chronic renal failure. Nephrol Dial Transplant 2004;19(8):2130–2.

77. Shiraishi N, Kitamura K, Miyoshi T, et al. Successful treatment of a patient with severe calcific uremic arteriolopathy (calciphylaxis) by etidronate disodium. Am J Kidney Dis 2006;48(1):151–4.

78. Hanafusa T, Yamaguchi Y, Tani M, et al. Intractable wounds caused by calcific uremic arteriolopathy treated with bisphosphonates. J Am Acad Dermatol 2007; 57(6):1021–5.

79. Byrnes CA, Shepler BM. Cinacalcet: a new treatment for secondary hyperparathyroidism in patients receiving hemodialysis. Pharmacotherapy 2005;25(5): 709–16.

80. Sharma A, Burkitt-Wright E, Rustom R. Cinacalcet as an adjunct in the successful treatment of calciphylaxis. Br J Dermatol 2006;155(6):1295–7.

81. Velasco N, MacGregor MS, Innes A, et al. Successful treatment of calciphylaxis with cinacalcet—an alternative to parathyroidectomy? Nephrol Dial Transplant 2006;21(7):1999–2004.

82. Brucculeri M, Cheigh J, Bauer G, et al. Long-term intravenous sodium thiosulfate in the treatment of a patient with calciphylaxis. Semin Dial 2005;18(5):431–4.

83. Hayden MR, Tyagi SC, Kolb L, et al. Vascular ossification-calcification in metabolic syndrome, type 2 diabetes mellitus, chronic kidney disease, and calciphylaxis-calcific uremic arteriolopathy: the emerging role of sodium thiosulfate. Cardiovasc Diabetol 2005;4(1):4.

84. Guerra G, Shah RC, Ross EA. Rapid resolution of calciphylaxis with intravenous sodium thiosulfate and continuous venovenous haemofiltration using low calcium replacement fluid: case report. Nephrol Dial Transplant 2005;20(6): 1260–2.

85. Hafner J, Keusch G, Wahl C, et al. Uremic small-artery disease with medial calcification and intimal hyperplasia (so-called calciphylaxis): a complication of chronic renal failure and benefit from parathyroidectomy. J Am Acad Dermatol 1995;33(6):954–62.

86. Arch-Ferrer JE, Beenken SW, Rue LW, et al. Therapy for calciphylaxis: an outcome analysis. Surgery 2003;134(6):941–4 [discussion: 944–5].

87. Dereure O, Leray H, Barneon G, et al. Extensive necrotizing livedo reticularis in a patient with chronic renal failure, hyperparathyroidism and coagulation disorder: regression after subtotal parathyroidectomy. Dermatology 1996; 192(2):167–70.

88. Amdo TD, Welker JA. An approach to the diagnosis and treatment of cryofibrinogenemia. Am J Med 2004;116(5):332–7.

89. Nash JW, Ross P Jr, Neil Crowson A, et al. The histopathologic spectrum of cryofibrinogenemia in four anatomic sites. Skin, lung, muscle, and kidney. Am J Clin Pathol 2003;119(1):114–22.

90. Smith SB, Arkin C. Cryofibrinogenemia: incidence, clinical correlations, and a review of the literature. Am J Clin Pathol 1972;58(5):524–30.

91. Blain H, Cacoub P, Musset L, et al. Cryofibrinogenaemia: a study of 49 patients. Clin Exp Immunol 2000;120(2):253–60.

92. Falanga V, Kirsner RS, Eaglstein WH, et al. Stanozolol in treatment of leg ulcers due to cryofibrinogenaemia. Lancet 1991;338(8763):347–8.

93. Revenga F, Aguilar C, Gonzalez R, et al. Cryofibrinogenaemia with a good response to stanozolol. Clin Exp Dermatol 2000;25(8):621–3.

94. Copeman PW. Cryofibrinogenaemia and skin ulcers: treatment with plasmapheresis. Br J Dermatol 1979;101(Suppl 17):57–8.

95. Kirsner RS, Eaglstein WH, Katz MH, et al. Stanozolol causes rapid pain relief and healing of cutaneous ulcers caused by cryofibrinogenemia. J Am Acad Dermatol 1993;28(1):71–4.

96. Rubegni P, Flori ML, Fimiani M, et al. A case of cryofibrinogenaemia responsive to stanozolol. Br J Haematol 1996;93(1):217–9.

97. Williamson AE, Cone LA, Huard GS 2nd. Spontaneous necrosis of the skin associated with cryofibrinogenemia, cryoglobulinemia, and homocystinuria. Ann Vasc Surg 1996;10(4):365–9.

98. Chartier M, Falanga V. Healing of ulcers due to cryofibrinogenemia with colchicine and high-dose pentoxifylline. Am J Clin Dermatol 2009;10(1):39–42.

99. Braverman IM. Skin signs of systemic disease. 3rd edition. Philadelphia: W.B. Saunders; 1997.

100. Peyri J, Moreno A, Marcoval J. Necrobiosis lipoidica. Semin Cutan Med Surg 2007;26(2):87–9.

101. Zeichner JA, Stern DW, Lebwohl M. Treatment of necrobiosis lipoidica with the tumor necrosis factor antagonist etanercept. J Am Acad Dermatol 2006; 54(3 Suppl 2):S120–1.

102. Noz KC, Korstanje MJ, Vermeer BJ. Ulcerating necrobiosis lipoidica effectively treated with pentoxifylline. Clin Exp Dermatol 1993;18(1):78–9.

103. Harth W, Linse R. Topical tacrolimus in granuloma annulare and necrobiosis lipoidica. Br J Dermatol 2004;150(4):792–4.

104. Reinhard G, Lohmann F, Uerlich M, et al. Successful treatment of ulcerated necrobiosis lipoidica with mycophenolate mofetil. Acta Derm Venereol 2000;80(4):312–3.

105. Stinco G, Parlangeli ME, De Francesco V, et al. Ulcerated necrobiosis lipoidica treated with cyclosporin A. Acta Derm Venereol 2003;83(2):151–3.

106. Stanway A, Rademaker M, Newman P. Healing of severe ulcerative necrobiosis lipoidica with cyclosporin. Australas J Dermatol 2004;45(2):119–22.

107. De Rie MA, Sommer A, Hoekzema R, et al. Treatment of necrobiosis lipoidica with topical psoralen plus ultraviolet A. Br J Dermatol 2002;147(4):743–7.

108. Durupt F, Dalle S, Debarbieux S, et al. Successful treatment of necrobiosis lipoidica with antimalarial agents. Arch Dermatol 2008;144(1):118–9.

109. Miura Y, Ardenghy M, Ramasastry S, et al. Coumadin necrosis of the skin: report of four patients. Ann Plast Surg 1996;37(3):332–7.

110. Chan YC, Valenti D, Mansfield AO, et al. Warfarin induced skin necrosis. Br J Surg 2000;87(3):266–72.

111. Ward CT, Chavalitanonda N. Atypical warfarin-induced skin necrosis. Pharmacotherapy 2006;26(8):1175–9.

112. Wynn SS, Jin DK, Essex DW. Warfarin-induced skin necrosis occurring four days after discontinuation of warfarin. Haemostasis 1997;27(5):246–50.

113. Franson TR, Rose HD, Spivey MR, et al. Late-onset, warfarin-caused necrosis occurring in a patient with infectious mononucleosis. Arch Dermatol 1984; 120(7):927–31.

114. DeFranzo AJ, Marasco P, Argenta LC. Warfarin-induced necrosis of the skin. Ann Plast Surg 1995;34(2):203–8.

115. Tai CY, Ierardi R, Alexander JB. A case of warfarin skin necrosis despite enoxaparin anticoagulation in a patient with protein S deficiency. Ann Vasc Surg 2004;18(2):237–42.

116. Rose VL, Kwaan HC, Williamson K, et al. Protein C antigen deficiency and warfarin necrosis. Am J Clin Pathol 1986;86(5):653–5.

117. Nazarian RM, Van Cott EM, Zembowicz A, et al. Warfarin-induced skin necrosis. J Am Acad Dermatol 2009;61(2):325–32.

118. Hunter JB, Lonsdale RJ, Wenham PW, et al. Heparin induced thrombosis: an important complication of heparin prophylaxis for thromboembolic disease in surgery. BMJ 1993;307(6895):53–5.

119. Warkentin TE, Elavathil LJ, Hayward CP, et al. The pathogenesis of venous limb gangrene associated with heparin-induced thrombocytopenia. Ann Intern Med 1997;127(9):804–12.

Complex Wounds and Their Management

Habeeba Park, MD[a], Carol Copeland, MD[a], Sharon Henry, MD[b], Adrian Barbul, MD[a,c],*

KEYWORDS

- Complex wound • Necrotizing fasciitis • Ischemia • Dressing

Complex wounds present a challenge to both the surgeon and patient in operative management, long-term care, cosmetic outcome, and effects on lifestyle, self-image, and general health. Although there is no single universally accepted definition, the term complex wound generally describes wounds that may anatomically involve multiple tissues, often develop after devastating injuries, and frequently do not heal in a timely manner or fail to heal completely. Comorbidities are common and often multiple. Complete healing often requires the use of advanced wound care techniques and/or products. Prolonged wound management times can delay chemoradiation treatments, extract a significant toll on patients' quality of life, compound psychological devastation on top of injury and illness, and may lead to cosmetically unacceptable results.[1]

RISK FACTORS

Commonly, each patient with complex wounds presents with multiple risk factors for their development. Immunocompromised patients, such as those with diabetes, human immunodeficiency virus infection, and sickle cell anemia and those receiving chemotherapy or other immunosuppressive therapy, are more prone to developing complex wounds than patients with normal immune function. Diabetic patients present a unique situation in which the combination of immunosuppression, poor vascular supply, and impaired neurologic function synergistically delays the healing process. Smoking causes vasoconstriction, inhibiting the delivery of nutrients and oxygen to regenerating tissues, and is often the main cause of arteriosclerosis. Other conditions that affect blood flow and nutrient delivery include obesity, tissue edema,

---

[a] Department of Surgery, Sinai Hospital of Baltimore, 2401 West Belvedere Avenue, Baltimore, MD 21215, USA
[b] Department of Surgery, Shock Trauma Center, University of Maryland Medical Center, Baltimore, MD 21201, USA
[c] Department of Surgery, Johns Hopkins Medical Institutions, Baltimore, MD, USA
* Corresponding author. Department of Surgery, Sinai Hospital of Baltimore, 2401 West Belvedere Avenue, Baltimore, MD 21215.
E-mail address: abarbul@jhmi.edu

Surg Clin N Am 90 (2010) 1181–1194
doi:10.1016/j.suc.2010.08.001
0039-6109/10/$ – see front matter © 2010 Elsevier Inc. All rights reserved.

surgical.theclinics.com

and peripheral arterial disease. Obesity is often accompanied by diabetes or peripheral vascular disease but by itself can cause dependent stress on lower body wounds because of sheer weight, leading to reduced blood flow and increased risk of ischemia, dehiscence, and infection. Other risk factors for poor wound healing include trauma, older age, obesity, alcoholism, and malnutrition.

Etiology

The causes of complex wounds span a wide variety of physical insults. Surgical wounds may heal poorly and can lead to a long-term nonhealing situation, which occurs most commonly in conjunction with risk factors such as inadequate surgical closure, ischemia, anastomotic failure, and infection. Other common mechanisms involve blunt or penetrating traumatic injuries with large and complex defects. The introduction of foreign material into wounds through penetration by bullets, projectiles, or penetrating objects increases the risk of infection and necrosis.

Complex, open orthopedic injuries often require advanced and challenging reconstructive techniques. The additional soft tissue injury can complicate primary repair and adds to the risk of infection. The initial assessment of such patients should include an evaluation to identify and correct life-threatening injuries and the resuscitation of the patient with correction of hypotension, hypoxemia, hypothermia, and coagulopathy. Assessment and treatment of open fractures is best performed concurrently with the general resuscitation of the patient. Early collaboration between the orthopedic and vascular teams can improve outcomes.

Both blunt and penetrating traumas may produce injury to a larger anatomic zone by direct tissue destruction and microvascular injury. There are 3 zones of injury: zone of necrosis, zone of stasis (adjacent to the zone of necrosis and extremely vulnerable to necrosis), and zone of hyperemia (outside the zone of stasis with viable tissue). With aggressive debridement of nonviable tissue, bacteriologic control, and fluid resuscitation, the zones, which are not defined in the acute setting, can be supported and allowed to demarcate.[2]

In penetrating trauma, damage is caused by several mechanisms such as laceration, crush, shock waves, and cavitation.[2] A high-velocity bullet disrupts structures well away from its path through the transfer of kinetic energy. Secondary missiles created from fragmented bone cause further destruction. Clothing and other contaminants may be sucked into the wound, increasing contamination and the risk of subsequent infection, which frequently results in tissue loss greater than that produced by the missile path. The magnitude of energy imparted by the concentrated spread of a shot causes high-impact shearing forces, leading to significant disruption of soft tissues, fractures and angulation of long bones, and piercing of vessels or indirectly causing vascular tears at fixation points.[3] With treatment of a mangled extremity, attempts to salvage an irreparably damaged extremity may condemn the patient to a protracted series of anesthetizations and operations, prolonged hospitalization, and eventually the disappointment of an insensate and possibly septic limb requiring amputation, delaying rehabilitation. The Mangled Extremity Severity Score (**Table 1**) for determining the ability or futility of extremity repair is one of a variety of scoring systems used by surgeons to treat traumatic extremities[4]; however, to date, there is no solid evidence supporting the use of these scoring systems. Although amputation at a level of normal tissue is indicated, functional outcome should be the priority in assessing for length.[5]

The phenomenon of reperfusion injury is important in the management of complex wounds, particularly in traumatic extremities. The failure of local antioxidant scavenging systems in the face of overwhelming oxidant production is associated with oxidative stress injury. The cascade of potent vasoactive eicosanoids, such as

Table 1
Mangled Extremity Severity Score

Criteria	Points
Skeletal/Soft Tissue Injury	
Low energy (stab, simple fracture, pistol GSW)	1
Medium energy (open or multiple fractures, dislocation)	2
High energy (high-speed MVA or rifle GSW)	3
Very high energy (high-speed trauma + gross contamination)	4
Limb Ischemia	
Pulse reduced or absent but perfusion normal	1[a]
Pulseless, paresthesias, diminished capillary refill	2
Cool, paralyzed, insensate, numb	3[a]
Shock	
Systolic BP always >90 mm Hg	0
Hypotensive transiently	1
Persistent hypotension	2
Age (y)	
<30	0
30–50	1
>50	2

A score >7 predicts a low likelihood of limb/extremity viability (>91% of patients will experience limb loss).[40]

Abbreviations: BP, blood pressure; GSW, gunshot wound; MVA, motor vehicle accident.

[a] Score doubled for ischemia >6 hours.

thromboxane A_2 and leukotriene B4, have both local and systemic proinflammatory effects. Local recruitment, activation, and sequestration of neutrophils also release oxygen reactive species and proteases, further compounding reperfusion injury. The systemic inflammatory response syndrome affects cytokine release, which affects the liver, lungs, bowel, heart, brain, and kidneys, leading to multiple organ dysfunction syndrome and usually resulting in fatality.[3] Prevention of ischemia and compartment syndrome reduces the risk of reperfusion injury.

Wound Infection

Infected wounds, either traumatic or surgical, heal poorly. Puncture wounds are associated with high infection rates because they involve deep inoculation of pathogens. Wounds contaminated with human or animal fecal contaminants have a high risk of infection despite therapeutic intervention.[6] Bite wounds are often underestimated because of early benign appearance. Human bite wounds are often infected with multiple organisms, including β-hemolytic streptococci, *Staphylococcus aureus, Staphylococcus epidermis, Corynebacterium, Eikenella corrodens, Bacteroides* sp, *Fusobacterium*, and *Clostridium*. Animal bites have the potential to cause significant wounds because of crushing and avulsion.[2] Antitetanus immune globulin and broad-spectrum antibiotics against aerobic and anaerobic organisms should be administered adhering to local protocols.[3]

Massive Soft Tissue Infection

Massive soft tissue infections include necrotizing fasciitis, gas gangrene, and Fournier gangrene. Necrotizing fasciitis is a rare, potentially lethal bacterial infection characterized by widespread necroses of the skin, subcutaneous tissue, and superficial fascia.[7] This fulminant disease can occur in almost any anatomic area, spreading along fascial planes, but primarily involves the superficial layers of the extremities, abdomen, or perineum as in Fournier gangrene. Patients may present with locally contained infections or septicemia, leading to multiple organ failure and death. Common symptoms include edema, skin induration, bullae, purulence, fluctuance, local warmth, pain out of proportion to the appearance of the skin lesion, and most significantly, tissue crepitus suggesting gas in the tissues.[7]

The gold standard for establishing the diagnosis of necrotizing fasciitis is encountering fascial necrosis and/or loss of tissue plane integrity found during surgical exploration. Tissues may demonstrate grayish pus and necrotic fascia, lack of bleeding, and lack of resistance to blunt dissection with the finger test, in which a probe or finger can be used to bluntly dissect down along the fascial planes. These infections are often polymicrobial. Major culprits include group A streptococcus, β-hemolytic streptococci, S aureus, Streptococcus viridians, coagulase-negative staphylococcus, Clostridium, Bacteroides sp, Escherichia coli, and Proteus. Prompt diagnosis and surgical intervention are key to patient survival because the infection spreads rapidly and carries a significant mortality. The progression of the disease can be fulminant, and any delay on the part of the patient or the treating team can have dire consequences. Serial debridements are frequently required, often in conjunction with the use of hyperbaric oxygen treatment. Thorough removal of all necrotic tissues offers the best hope of rapid source control. Irrigation of the wound bed at the time of debridement decreases the bacterial count and limits the spread of the disease. Colostomies may be necessary to divert stool away from wounds in abdominal and perineal causes. Early empirical antibiotics are chosen to cover gram-negative, gram-positive, and anaerobic bacteria. Cultures taken during surgical debridement allow the broad-spectrum antibiotics to be narrowed to the specific pathogens involved. Wounds are left open and dressed appropriately until they are clean and are candidates for secondary closure.[7] Some wounds are left to heal completely by secondary intention.

MANAGEMENT OF COMPLEX WOUNDS

The steps involved in complex wound treatment include (1) searching for and treatment of life-threatening trauma/conditions, (2) obtaining a thorough history and physical examination, (3) examining the wound using aseptic technique to prevent further contamination, (4) anesthetizing the wound before cleansing, (5) performing hair removal, skin disinfection, hemostasis, surgical debridement, and mechanical cleansing, and (6) use of antibiotics and drains and open wound management.[6] Prompt and thorough assessment and timely operative management are key to optimal treatment of complex wounds.

Assessment

The anatomic considerations in the assessment of complex wounds include the possibility of scarring around vital structures such as nerves and tendons. High-risk injuries, such as circumferential burns, crush injuries, and lacerations, can lead to vascular compromise.[5] The initial assessment should include advanced trauma life support evaluation to identify and correct life-threatening injuries and resuscitation of the patient, including correction of hypotension, hypoxemia, hypothermia, and coagulopathy. Assessment and treatment of open fractures is best performed concurrently with the general resuscitation of the patient.

Important history points to investigate include mechanism of injury and magnitude of energy imparted, entrapment or prolonged extrication, and hypotension, all of which can increase the incidence of compartment syndrome. Advanced age or patient history of smoking and diabetes contribute to poor outcomes and may necessitate treatment modifications.[8–10]

Physical examination should include an examination of the wound, circumferential examination of the limb, and a detailed neurovascular examination. Absent plantar sensation should be documented but is no longer considered an indication for amputation in the mangled extremity. Gross correction of limb deformity and shortening with splinting may result in correction of kinking and spasm of many compromised vascular trees and should be attempted before undertaking more advanced vascular evaluations, such as ankle brachial indices, angiography, or computed tomographic (CT) angiography. Radiographic evaluation should include imaging of the affected area including the joint above and below the injury.

Vascular status should be determined through assessment of pulses, examination of capillary refill and skin temperature, Doppler examination, noninvasive vascular studies for vessel competence, neurovascular monitoring, Doppler cutaneous mapping, or angiography/arteriography.[5,11] However, preoperative angiography should be avoided if a delay in the angiography suite is anticipated[3] or if the patient is in extremis. Palpation of the bone adjacent to a traumatic wound may detect tenderness or instability consistent with an underlying bony injury,[6] necessitating further workup or orthopedic intervention. Plain radiographs, CT, or magnetic resonance imaging are used to assess the presence of foreign bodies or possible osteomyelitis.[12] The most widely used classification system for open fractures is the Anderson and Gustilo classification (**Table 2**).[13,14] Wound size, fracture comminution, periosteal stripping, contamination, and vascular compromise are taken into consideration. The classification is best assigned after surgical debridement to avoid underestimation of the extent of soft tissue damage.

Antibiotics

Antibiotic therapy needs to begin in the emergency room and should include a broad-spectrum antibiotic, such as cefazolin. Single-antibiotic therapy with ciprofloxacin has been shown to be efficacious for Gustilo types I and II fractures but not for type III fractures.[15] Penicillin and an aminoglycoside are imperative in grossly contaminated wounds to avoid gram-negative and clostridial sepsis. Tetanus toxoid should be administered if the patient's immunization status is not current, with tetanus immune

Table 2	
Anderson and Gustilo classification of open fractures	
Type of Fracture	**Characteristics**
Type I	Wound <2 cm, no significant comminution/stripping/contamination
Type II	Wound 2–10 cm, no significant comminution/stripping/contamination
Type III	Wound >10 cm, extensive comminution/stripping/contamination
Type IIIA	Local tissues sufficient to close the wound
Type IIIB	Local tissues insufficient for closure; tissue transfers may be required for closure
Type IIIC	Local tissues insufficient for closure; vascular repair/reconstruction necessary

Data from Gustilo RB, Anderson JT. Prevention of infection in the treatment of one thousand and twenty-five open fractures of long bones. J Bone Joint Surg Am 1976;58(4):453–8.

globulin being added when there are high-risk wounds and the immunization history is unknown.

Skeletal Stabilization

Skeletal stabilization may involve initial provisional external fixation for damage control in the face of multiple trauma or vascular injury or for allowing soft tissue stabilization with aggressive debridement. Locked reamed intramedullary nailing is now possible for many metaphyseal and diaphyseal fractures because of advancements in nailing technologies and affords earlier weight bearing and minimal additional surgical trauma to the limb with improved union rates.[16] Techniques for periarticular plating have also advanced, and many fractures are now fixed with less-invasive approaches for meta-diaphyseal reconstruction while still allowing anatomic reduction of articular surfaces.

Revascularization

In some studies, early shunting of both artery and vein in both penetrating and blunt injuries reduces the need for fasciotomy and causes a significant decrease in the incidence of contracture and amputation. Arterial injury and arrest of distal inflow results in tissue hypoperfusion, which is further aggravated by hypovolemic shock and generalized vasoconstriction. Striated muscle tolerates warm ischemia for only 6 to 8 hours depending on the level of injury and availability of collateral flow. Soft tissue injury is further compounded by the phenomenon of ischemia-reperfusion injury. Vascular injuries are present in 10% to 48% of cases of complex limb trauma, and the amputation rates in this group are as high as 85%.[3]

SURGICAL MANAGEMENT

Surgical therapy remains the cornerstone for treating deep-plane tissue infection and traumatic injuries.[12] This therapy is effective in controlling bacterial burden; removing foreign bodies, debris, and nonviable tissue; and creating a sterile, well-vascularized, healthy wound bed amenable to primary closure or other surgical coverage. The principles of management involve assessing the patient's clinical status and the wound itself, appropriate timing of intervention, providing antibiotic therapy when necessary, and planning and executing surgical therapy, including the establishment of a clean wound bed and closure/reconstructive strategies. For the acute traumatic wound, the "golden period" has been defined as 6 to 24 hours from the time of injury, based on laboratory and clinical studies on the doubling time of bacteria, with progression to an invasive infection, and from clinical outcomes demonstrating decreased risk for infection after debridement during that period.[2] High-energy trauma, either penetrating or blunt, meriting the term complex, is characterized by considerable damage to all structures. The main artery and vein and long vessel segments may be crushed, punctured, and possibly denuded of the adjacent viable muscle and soft tissue. The typical features of a high-energy trauma are damage and loss of muscle and soft tissue, disruption of collateral vessels, high-pressure hematomas, nerve injury, and varying degrees of wound contamination.[3]

Debridement

The first steps in surgical management of a complex wound are debridement and hemostasis. Establishing a clean wound is essential; often wounds require debridement of necrotic bone and/or soft tissue. Debridement and immediate closure of the acute wound in one step is the main goal for selected wounds without intrinsic, mechanical, or extrinsic deficiency; however, serial debridement is important when there is an inability to accurately assess the amount of nonviable tissue or the extent of debridement required at the initial operation.[2] Tissue tension, postoperative edema, and swelling lead to increased ischemia at suture lines, resulting in necrosis and dehiscence.[11] Placement of dependent drains helps obliterate potential spaces, helping wound closure and preventing potential wound infections from fluid collections. Initially, partial-thickness wound defects can be managed conservatively with wet-to-wet dressings, oral antibiotics, and local wound debridement; however, if superficial debridement continues to progress, early aggressive soft tissue reconstruction should be performed.[11]

Debridement with orthopedic injuries was once considered emergent; however, more recently this tenet has come under some scrutiny. Although debridement performed less than 5 hours from injury is associated with a significant decrease in infection, it is often logistically difficult in the patient with multiple trauma. The majority of current literature suggests no obvious advantage to performing surgical debridement within 6 hours after injury versus doing so between 6 and 24 hours after injury; the benefits of delay greater than 6 hours include better patient resuscitation and coordination of resources. There is no support for elective (>24 hours delay) debridement of open fractures.[17-19]

In tissue assessment, a "4C" guideline for viability of muscle has been described: color, consistency, contraction, and circulation.[6] These clinical indicators of viability are more accurate when the wound is examined several days after the initial wound repair.[6] Wound exploration includes defining the zone of injury, identifying the key anatomic structures, and defining the extent of infection or necrosis. The consensus among experts is wide and aggressive surgical excision, assessment of skin and tissue vascularity, and subsequent appropriate debridement of devascularized tissues. At the skin and subcutaneous level, edges need to be examined for vascularity and the amount of undermining.[2] If there is significant degloving, necrosis, or infection, serial excisions can be considered before reconstruction.[20] With traumatic orthopedic injury, skeletal integrity should be restored to ensure the safety of subsequent vascular repairs, including timely internal or external fixation before definitive repairs of artery and vein are performed.[3] On completion of vascular repairs, fasciotomy should be performed in patients with delayed admission, significant edema, raised compartment pressures, and discernable drift toward plantar flexion of the foot.[3]

In traumatic orthopedic injuries, time to debridement is no longer considered a risk factor for the development of infection. The Lower Extremity Amputation Prevention (LEAP) study, a multicenter, prospective, observational study of 315 patients with severe high-energy lower extremity injuries, reported that 84 patients (27%) developed an infection within the first 3 months after the injury. There were no significant differences between patients who developed an infection and those who did not when they were compared with regard to the time from the injury to the first debridement, the time from admission to the first debridement, or the time from the first debridement to soft tissue coverage. The time between the injury and admission to the definitive trauma treatment center was an independent predictor of the likelihood of infection.[19]

Aggressive mechanical debridement of open fractures should proceed systematically, working from outside to inside, with longitudinal extensions to allow debridement of deeper tissues while protecting soft tissue coverage of vital structures and bone, where possible. Delivery of bone ends into the wound for curettage is necessary to remove retained foreign bodies. Any devitalized tissue should be removed. Pressure irrigation with saline or soap solution is recommended. Antibiotic solutions are associated with more wound infections and add cost, potential immunologic sensitization, and selection of resistant organisms.

Compartment Release

Several factors increase the risk of extremity compartment syndrome, including traumatic energy imparted to the wound, segmental injuries to the limb, systemic hypotension, hypoxemia, and coagulopathy. A heightened index of suspicion in high-energy mechanisms and patients who are unstable helps to avoid missed or late diagnosis, which leads to renal and systemic complications, such as rhabdomyolysis, infection, amputation, or Volkmann ischemic contracture. Intracompartment pressure is measured with a standard arterial line pressure transducer system or with portable devices, such as the Stryker STIK catheter (Stryker Orthopaedics, Mahwah, NJ, USA). Intracompartment pressure within 30 mm Hg of the diastolic blood pressure indicates compartment syndrome and is considered the threshold for fasciotomy.[21] Principles of compartment release include wide release of all compartments, leaving the skin open, incorporation of traumatic wounds in the fasciotomy, maintenance of a wide soft tissue bridge over the tibia, and preservation of venous drainage.[22] Full decompression of the deep posterior compartment of the leg is imperative to preserve ankle function and protect plantar sensation.

Wound Irrigation

Although the use of high-pressure irrigation decreases the bacterial load and debrides traumatized tissues, it does contribute to the development of postoperative edema; therefore, this modality should be reserved for contaminated wounds.[6] Irrigation via high-pressure systems, pulsatile flow, or other modalities should be used in conjunction with sharp surgical debridement for wounds with a large bacterial load. A newer method is Hydrocision (Hydrocision Inc, North Billerica, MA, USA), which simultaneously cuts and removes tissues with water through a high-pressure opening. This method is particularly useful in concavities and tight spaces, and has been used successfully, particularly in the debridement of burns.[2] Normal saline is recommended, emphasizing the mechanical effect of irrigation as opposed to the antibacterial activity of any more potent solutions, which may lead to irritation. Insufficient cleansing or excision allows gram-positive and gram-negative organisms to initiate cellulitis and even progress to necrotizing fasciitis or gas gangrene.[3]

Dressings

Tissues should not be allowed to desiccate because desiccation results in cell death, necrosis, infection, edema, and can lead to further soft tissue destruction.[11] Splinting should involve good padding to avoid heel decubiti. Rigid circumferential dressings should be avoided. Moist wound healing has been shown to facilitate epithelialization, promote angiogenesis, and decrease pain during dressing changes. Film dressings are adhesive waterproof dressings, which can be used as primary or secondary dressings that allow wound visualization. Foams, alginates, and hydrofibers are types of dressings that absorb excess exudates, promote moist wound healing, and provide insulation and protection from further traumatic injury.[12] Some dressings are silver-impregnated, promoting an antibacterial environment and decreasing colonization. The use of topical antimicrobials, such as triple antibiotic ointment, has been implicated as a major source of contact dermatitis and possible pseudomonas overgrowth, so their use should be limited.[12] The use of antimicrobial creams containing malic acid or hypochlorite solutions (Dakin solution) decrease bacterial colonization but can cause inflammation of surrounding tissue, impede capillary blood flow to granulating tissue, or damage fibroblasts, causing impairment in healing. Wounds can be packed with gauze wet dressings and reassessed for potential serial redebridement. Serial dressing changes are usually necessary until a granulating wound bed becomes evident. Presence of residual necrotic tissue, foreign bodies, or infection demands additional meticulous operative debridements.[6]

Negative Pressure Wound Therapy

Until the introduction of the vacuum-assisted closure (V. A. C. Therapy © Kinetic Concepts Inc, San Antonia, TX, USA) device, the principal modality of treatment involved packing and dressing changes to promote healing by secondary intention.[1] Negative pressure wound therapy (NPWT) has dramatically changed the surgical approach and time to heal a wide variety of complex and difficult wounds. The NPWT device provides a close to ideal environment for temporizing coverage. This device provides a moist environment and promotes and accelerates the growth of healthy granulation tissue while decreasing the presence of infectious agents. NPWT has been used effectively in a variety of wounds, including open abdominal wounds, wounds of lower extremities, pressure wounds/decubitus ulcers, and exposed bone.[1] NPWT can be used as a longer-term dressing in candidates who do not undergo surgery, allowing for wound control until the patients are stable enough to undergo a definitive closure. Some studies have shown that its use has decreased the need for secondary amputations.[23] In the open abdominal wound, NPWT decreases the incidence of abdominal compartment syndrome, protects and contains the abdominal contents, avoids the need for fascial sutures, and exerts a mechanical pull on the wound edges, resisting the unopposed pull of the oblique muscles. Thus the abdominal wall is pulled together, leading to a higher rate of successful fascial closure. It has been claimed that the microdeformational forces of the open-pore foam stimulate cell division and proliferation, promoting angiogenesis and granulation, and decrease matrix metalloproteinases, which normally act to degrade the extracellular matrix; however, the superiority of sponge or gauze as part of an NPWT has neither been studied nor established. NPWT also acts to remove excess fluid and promote wound contraction.[23] NPWT should be discontinued on excessive bleeding, wound sepsis, or hemodynamic compromise (when used in the chest) or if the wound shows no signs of improvement over a prolonged period.[23]

RECONSTRUCTION

Once the infection is controlled and viable tissue defined, treatment progresses to wound coverage, including direct primary closure and free flaps or other complex reconstruction.[12] In terms of coverage, a reconstructive ladder algorithm can be applied. The first step on the ladder is to allow the wound to form granulation tissue and "heal from the inside out." Disadvantages include prolonged healing time, dressing changes, suboptimal scar, and prolonged immobility of adjacent joints. If possible, primary closure is performed; disadvantages of primary closure include potential wound infection and the need for advanced surgical technique to repair involved structures.[2] In some wounds, delayed primary closure after a second look 48 to 72 hours after the initial operative intervention may be necessary. For scar minimization, W- and Z-plasties may be used, decreasing tensions per length of the wound.[6] Secondary intention healing can also be allowed depending on the size of the wound, the presence of infection, or the preservation of dermal elements.[11]

Skin substitutes, with properties of adherence to the wound bed, elasticity, pliability, and flexibility, maintain a barrier to microfloral invasion, help with wound fluid balance, and retain integrity over time. These substitutes serve as a nonsurgical option for patients with high surgical risk or when tissue options are limited or compromised by injury.[12] Placement of skin graft requires a clean viable wound bed, hemostasis, and appropriate dressings to protect the graft.[2] Human skin allograft can enhance healing of wounds that would be normally left open because of significant tissue loss, contamination, chronicity, or questionable secondary closure or closure with autograft. In contaminated wounds, allograft has the advantage of adhering to the wound, conferring the benefits of early wound closure, promoting vascularization and resistance to infection. Allograft can be used to test for potential autograft take.[24] Disadvantages of allografts include need for meticulous wound bed preparation, potential poor esthetics, contour defects, and poor durability.[2]

More advanced surgical techniques are local tissue rearrangement or use of local flaps, including fasciocutaneous flaps, musculocutaneous flaps, fascial flaps with skin graft, and composite flaps with bone and skin, which include their own blood supply and provide tissue durability. However, these techniques require a more complex operation and a small zone of injury, which does not include the flap to be elevated.[2] Selection of local versus distant flaps are based on the presence of infection, defect depth, presence/absence of vascular supply, and damage to other bodily areas, precluding the use of local flaps.[11] Tissue mobilization is limited by the history of radiation therapy, bacterial colonization and contamination, delayed healing from other wounds, and pressure from lying and sitting.[25] It is important to assess for existing hernias and previous surgeries, which may have compromised tissue blood supply,[25] particularly in considering abdominal tissue coverage for pelvic wounds. Whole muscle harvest is used to maximize the number of perforating blood vessels, bringing in new blood supply, and helps the area to heal.[25] Because muscle flaps are bulky, fill large defects, obliterate dead space, are malleable, and are well vascularized, they are considered the gold standard.[2] Free tissue transfer from remote sites with revascularization at the reconstructive site using microsurgical techniques[25] can allow for a one-step operation of the most complex wounds and more freedom in reconstruction in areas where local flaps are not available. There is, however, a potential for tissue loss as a result of vascular anastomotic failure.[2] Flaps should be assessed frequently for viability, tension from edema, and development of necrosis. The anterolateral thigh flap holds great promise for lower extremity reconstruction because it may be used for coverage and the fascial component may be used for tendinous reconstruction.[26] Osteomyocutaneous transplants from the iliac crest or the fibula (composite flaps) can bring vascularized tissue into a large combined soft tissue and bone defect.

After skeletal stabilization, staged soft tissue reconstruction may be necessary in orthopedic injuries. When possible, the primary closure of open fractures in grade II and IIIA fractures may decrease the risk of infection.[27] Dead space management to decrease infection risk can be facilitated by the use of antibiotic-impregnated polymethylmethacrylate bead pouches with significantly decreased infection rates.[28] NPWT also isolates the wound from the hospital and intensive care unit (ICU) flora with no documented benefit with respect to infection rates but clear improvements in patient tolerance, work intensity, and cost.[29] NPWT should be avoided in patients with coagulopathy because of the risk of bleeding; furthermore, circumferential wrapping of the extremity with NPWT is not recommended because excessive pressure may develop, leading to skin breakdown or compartment syndrome.

Bony Reconstruction

Multiple techniques for bony reconstruction exist and include extensive autogenous grafting or bone transport with distraction osteogenesis techniques.[30] Recent advances using the patients' own tissues include alternative bone graft harvesting techniques, such as the Reamer-Irrigator-Aspirator system (Synthes, Paoli, PA, USA). Biologically active adjuncts, such as platelet-derived growth factors or synthetic recombinant human bone morphogenetic protein (rhBMP) (Wyeth, Andover, MA, USA), can improve outcome and reduce nonunion and reoperation rates with fractures.[31]

OUTCOMES

Operative technique is important in the prevention of soft tissue complications. Atraumatic technique such as the use of skin hooks and loupe magnification, hemostasis during exposure, use of drains, and postoperative dressings contribute to uncomplicated postoperative healing.[11] Abscess cavities should be drained adequately, and any infected, devitalized, or necrotic tissue should be debrided.[2]

Patient factors, such as diabetes and smoking, are well known to increase the risk of wound complications, infections, and nonunions.[8,9,32,33] Ultrasound bone stimulators and the prophylactic use of rhBMP in bony defects of open fractures can successfully counteract these effects.[34] Mortality in the elderly is as high as 33% in the first 12 months after an open tibia fracture; amputation may be preferable to salvage in this age group.[10] Ambulation is encouraged starting on postoperative day 1 when possible; if the patient is bed-bound, low-pressure beds and frequent turning is recommended to avoid pressure necrosis.[25] However, there are a few reports on long-term outcomes and rehabilitation of patients who survive massive soft tissue infections such as necrotizing fasciitis; more research is needed in these populations.

Compartment syndrome and increasing Gustillo and Anderson type open fractures are associated with increased complications.[13,18,35] Neurovascular injury, amount of bone loss, type of bacterial contamination, and presence of deep soft tissue defects have also been associated with a high incidence of infection.[35,36] Aggressive management with fasciotomies, soft tissue reconstruction, and early prophylactic bone grafting are important in minimizing long-term disability. Sepsis in type IIIB open fractures was 52% in 1984; current rates with aggressive staged management are between 17% and 27%.[13,18,19]

The Anderson and Gustilo classification system has successfully correlated with outcomes such as nonunion, infection, and amputation.[13] These outcomes, however, have been shown to have only a 60% interobserver agreement at best.[37] Multiple scoring systems for assessment of the mangled extremity have been evaluated retrospectively.[38–40] When evaluated in a prospectively, the clinical utility of these scores is not demonstrated. The low sensitivity failed to support the validity of the scores as predictors of amputation.[41]

In cases of necrotizing fasciitis, there is little prior research done on long-term outcomes and no tools are validated for assessment of function. In a retrospective review of patients with necrotizing soft tissue infections at one institution over a 4-year period, involvement of an extremity was independently associated with a higher incidence of functional limitation. Other factors that were associated with functional limitation were higher Acute Physiology and Chronic Health Evaluation score, ICU days, and delay of therapy.[42] However, more prospective data and longitudinal follow-up are necessary to develop tools in measuring outcomes in patients with necrotizing fasciitis. The rate of mortality in this population has also been found to be significantly higher than population controls, with infections such as pneumonia, cholecystitis, and sepsis being major causes of death.[43] In a study of 345 patients, the average clinical follow-up was 3.3 years. Age was found to be the most important determinant of long-term survival. Patients who have had an episode of necrotizing soft tissue infection should be counseled, encouraged to modify other comorbid factors such as obesity, smoking, and diabetes, and long-term follow-up should be supported.

SUMMARY

Acute complex wounds present a unique challenge for surgeons. Good surgical technique, early appropriate surgical intervention, source control, early use of broad-spectrum antibiotic therapy, early tissue coverage, and avoidance of pressure on healing wounds help prevent postoperative complications and are the basis of treatment of complex wounds. V. A. C. Therapy has been shown to accelerate healing rates and is also economically efficient, less burdensome, and more patient-friendly than some of the other wet-to-dry dressings for large wounds.[1] Attention must also be given to preservation of function and maximization of functional outcomes for the patient in the treatment of complex wounds, particularly in patients with extremity involvement. More studies are necessary to further understand the effect on long-term functional outcomes.

REFERENCES

1. Stoeckel W, David L, Levine E, et al. Vacuum-assisted closure for the treatment of complex breast wounds. Breast 2006;15:610–3.
2. Lee CK, Hansen SL. Management of acute wounds. Surg Clin North Am 2009;89: 659–76.
3. Barros D'Sa AA, Harkin DW, Blair PH, et al. The Belfast approach to managing complex lower limb vascular injuries. Eur J Vasc Endovasc Surg 2006;32:246–56.
4. Togawa S, Yamami N, Nakayama H, et al. The validity of the mangled extremity severity score in the assessment of upper limb injuries. J Bone Joint Surg Br 2005;87(11):1516–9.
5. Sterling J, Gibran NS, Klein MB. Acute management of hand burns. Hand Clin 2009;25:453–9.
6. Edlich RF, Rodeheaver GT, Thacker JG, et al. Revolutionary advances in the management of traumatic wounds in the emergency department during the last 40 years: part I. J Emerg Med 2010;38(1):40–50.
7. Angoules AG, Kontakis G, Drakoulakis E, et al. Necrotising fasciitis of upper and lower limb: a systematic review. Injury 2007;38S:S18–25.
8. Hirose CB, Borelli J, Mitchell S, et al. Closed tibia fractures in patients with diabetes mellitus: complications and relative risk. In: Presented Orthopedic Trauma Association Annual Meeting. Salt Lake City (UT), October 9–11, 2003.
9. Harvey EJ, Agel J, Selznick HS, et al. Deleterious effect of smoking on healing of open tibial shaft fractures. Am J Orthop 2002;31:518–21.
10. Beauchamp N, Court-Brown CM. The early mortality rate of tibial fractures in the elderly. In: Presented Orthopedic Trauma Association Annual Meeting. Salt Lake City (UT), October 9–11, 2003.
11. Levin LS. Soft tissue coverage options for ankle wounds. Foot Ankle Clin 2001;6: 853–66.
12. Pozez A, Aboutanos S, Lucas V. Diagnosis and treatment of uncommon wounds. Clin Plast Surg 2007;34:749–64.
13. Gustillo RB, Anderson JT. Prevention of infection in the treatment of one thousand and twenty-five open fractures of long bones: retrospective and prospective analyses. J Bone Joint Surg Am 1976;58:453–8.

14. Gustilo RB, Mendoza RM, Williams DN. Problems in the management of type III (severe) open fractures: a new classification of type III open fractures. J Trauma 1984;24:742–6.

15. Patzakis MJ, Bains RS, Shepherd L, et al. Prospective, randomized, double blind study comparing single antibiotic agent, ciprofloxacin, to combination antibiotic therapy in open fracture wounds. J Orthop Trauma 2000;14(8):529–33.

16. Ziran B, Darowish M, Klatt BA, et al. Intramedullary nailing in open tibia fractures: a comparison of two techniques. Int Orthop 2004;28(4):235–8.

17. Werner CM, Pierpont Y, Pollak AN. The urgency of surgical debridement in the management of open fractures. J Am Acad Orthop Surg 2008;16:369–75.

18. Khatod M, Botte MJ, Hoyt DB, et al. Outcomes in open tibia fractures: relationship between delay in treatment and infection. J Trauma 2003;55(5):949–54.

19. Pollak AN, Jones AL, Castillo RC, et al, LEAP study group. The relationship between time to surgical debridement and incidence of infection after open high-energy lower extremity trauma. J Bone Joint Surg Am 2010;92:7–15.

20. Arnez ZM, Khan U, Tyler MP. Classification of soft tissue degloving in limb trauma. J Plast Reconstr Aesthet Surg 2009. DOI: 10.1016/j.bjps.2009.11.029.

21. McQueen MM, Court-Brown CM. Compartment monitoring in tibial fractures: the pressure threshold for decompression. J Bone Joint Surg Br 1996;78:99–104.

22. Sise M, Shackford S. Vascular trauma. Greenfield's surgery: scientific principles and practice. 4th edition. Philadelphia (PA): Lippencott Williams & Wilkins; 2005. Figure 27.4.

23. Parrett BM, Bayer LR, Orgill DP. Use of microdeformational wound therapy in difficult wounds. Operat Tech Gen Surg 2003;1524–153X/06. DOI: 10.1053/j.optechgensurg.2006.11.003.

24. Spence RJ, Wong L. The enhancement of wound healing with human skin allograft. Surg Clin North Am 1997;77(3):731–45.

25. Zenn M. Closure techniques for large pelvic wounds. Semin Colon Rectal Surg 2004;15:59–67.

26. Wei FC, Jain V, Celik N, et al. Have we found an ideal soft tissue flap? An experience with 672 anterolateral thigh flaps. Plast Reconstr Surg 2002;109(7):2219–26.

27. Delong WG, Born CT, Wie SY. Aggressive treatment of 119 open fracture wounds. J Trauma 1999;46:1049–54.

28. Ostermann PA, Seligson D, Henry SL. Local antibiotic therapy for severe open fractures. A review of 1085 consecutive cases. J Bone Joint Surg Br 1995; 77(1):93–7.

29. Bihariesingh VJ, Stolarczyk EM, Karim RB, et al. Plastic solutions for orthopedic problems. Arch Orthop Trauma Surg 2004;124:73–6.

30. Keeling JJ, Gwinn DE, Tintle SM, et al. Short-term outcomes of severe open wartime tibial fractures treated with ring external fixation. J Bone Joint Surg Am 2008;90:2643–51.

31. Jimenez ML, Anderson TL. The use of allograft, platelet derived growth factors, and internal bone stimulation for treatment of recalcitrant nonunions. In: Orthopedic Trauma Association Annual Meeting. Salt Lake City (UT), October 9–11, 2003.

32. Schmitz MA, Finnegan M, Natarajan R, et al. Effect of smoking on tibial shaft fracture healing. Clin Orthop 1999;1(365):184–200.

33. Castillo RC, Bosse MJ, MacKenzie EJ, et al. LEAP Study Group. Impact of smoking on fracture healing and risk of complications in limb-threatening open tibia fractures. J Orthop Trauma 2005;19:151–7.

34. Cook SD, Ryaby JP, McCabe J, et al. Acceleration of tibial and distal radius fracture healing in patients who smoke. Clin Orthop 1997;1(337):197–207.

35. Suedkamp NE, Barbey N, Veuskens A, et al. The incidence of osteitis in open fractures: an analysis of 948 open fractures (a review of the Hannover experience). J Orthop Trauma 1993;7(5):473–82.

36. Kreder HJ, Armstrong P. A review of open tibia fractures in children. J Pediatr Orthop 1995;15:482–8.

37. Brumback RJ, Jones AL. Interobserver agreement in the classification of open fractures of the tibia. The results of a survey of two hundred and forty-five orthopaedic surgeons. J Bone Joint Surg Am 1994;76(8):1162–6.

38. Howe HR, Poole GV, Hansen KJ, et al. Salvage of lower extremities following combined orthopaedic and vascular trauma. A predictive salvage index. Am Surg 1987;53(4):205–8.

39. Russell WL, Sailors DM, Whittle TB, et al. Limb salvage versus traumatic amputation: a decision based on a seven-part predictive index. Ann Surg 1991;213: 473–81.

40. Johansen K, Daines M, Howey T, et al. Objective criteria accurately predict amputation following lower extremity trauma. J Trauma 1990;30:568–73.

41. Bosse M, MacKenzie EJ, Kellam JF, et al. A prospective evaluation of the clinical utility of the lower extremity injury-severity scores. J Bone Joint Surg Am 2001;83: 3–14.

42. Pham T, Moore M, Costa BA, et al. Assessment of functional limitation after necrotizing soft tissue infection. J Burn Care Res 2009;30:301–6.

43. Light T, Choi K, Thomsen TA, et al. Long-term outcomes of patients with necrotizing fasciitis. J Burn Care Res 2010;31:93–9.

Medical and Surgical Therapy for Advanced Chronic Venous Insufficiency

Ronnie Word, MD

KEYWORDS

- Venous ulceration • Venous insufficiency • Venous ablation
- Venous reconstruction

Venous ulceration is the most serious consequence of chronic venous insufficiency. The disease has been known for more than 3.5 millennia with wound care centers established as early as 1500 BC.

Unfortunately, still today it is a very poorly managed medical condition by most physicians despite that a great deal has been learned about the pathogenesis and treatment for venous ulcerations. We find that many wound care clinics treat the wound and not the cause of the problem. In this article, we review the basic pathophysiology of advanced chronic venous insufficiency (CVI) and review the most up-to-date information with regard to medical therapy and different options of surgical therapy to address the underlying venous pathology responsible for chronic ulcers.

EPIDEMIOLOGY OF CHRONIC VENOUS DISORDERS AND VENOUS ULCERS

Most studies have shown that about 1% of the adult population has a history of a healed or open venous leg ulcer and in elderly patients older than 65 years the prevalence may increase up to 4%.[1]

In recent years, new epidemiologic studies have been published. The Bonn Vein Study from Germany[2] enrolled 3072 participants, ages 17 to 89 years. The study found that approximately 2.9% had advanced CVI with skin changes such as pigmentation or eczema and 0.7% had either a healed ulcer or an active venous leg ulcer.

Also, in a multicenter study of 40,095 adults in Poland,[3] advanced chronic venous disease with skin changes was found in 4.6%, healed venous ulcer in 1.0%, and an active ulcer in 0.5% of participants.

Department of Surgery, Marshfield Clinic, 1000 North Oak Avenue, Marshfield, WI 54449, USA
E-mail address: Word.ronnie@marshfieldclinic.org

Surg Clin N Am 90 (2010) 1195–1214
doi:10.1016/j.suc.2010.08.008
0039-6109/10/$ – see front matter © 2010 Published by Elsevier Inc.

surgical.theclinics.com

In one study[4] in the United States, it was found that the overall incidences of venous stasis syndrome and venous ulcer were 76.1 and 18.0 per 100,000 person-years, respectively.

CEAP CLASSIFICATION

For the practicing general surgeon to better understand and manage CVDs (chronic venous diseases) it is important to be familiar with the CEAP classification. This comprehensive classification system was created by an international ad hoc committee of the American Venous Forum (AVF) in 1994[5] to standardize the reporting and treatment of chronic venous disorders and to establish a framework in which the clinical manifestations found in CVD are paired with pathophysiologic mechanisms and anatomic locations of veins in the lower extremities.

The CEAP classification includes the clinical class (C), the etiology (E), the anatomic (A) distribution, and the underlying pathophysiology (P).

The following 7 clinical categories are recognized:

C_0 Limbs without venous disease
C_1 Telangiectasias
C_2 Varicose veins
C_3 Edema
C_4 Skin changes
      C_{4a} Pigmentation, eczema
      C_{4b} Lipodermatosclerosis, atrophie blanche
C_5 Healed venous stasis ulcer
C_6 Active venous stasis ulcer.

Underlying etiology is further classified as *primary,* which represents a degenerative process in the normally formed vessel walls and valves, without an identifiable mechanism of venous dysfunction. *Secondary* etiology results from an antecedent event, usually an episode of DVT that results in an acquired inflammatory destructive process. *Congenital* etiology represents malformation of the blood vessels. These are rare and not further detailed in this article.

The anatomic distribution refers to which venous segment is affected by CVD. The superficial vein refers to the saphenous systems, reticular and varicose veins, or whether the deep venous system or the perforating veins are involved.

The underlying pathophysiology is basically divided into 2 major categories: whether it is reflux or obstruction of the venous system.

PATHOPHYSIOLOGY OF SEVERE CVI

Current theories of the etiology of severe CVI relate to chronic venous hypertension, which leads to failure of vein valves and vein walls and an inflammatory response that leads to skin changes.[6,7] Abnormalities in the valves or lumen of the superficial deep and communicating (perforator) veins lead to persistent ambulatory venous hypertension.

In the superficial venous system, primary reflux attributable to valvular incompetence is the most frequent pathologic mechanism of venous hypertension. Evidence favors a weakness in the vein wall producing dilation with enlargement of the valve ring, preventing coaptation of the leaflets.[8] The perforating veins may also become primarily incompetent; however, a more typical scenario is to have a saphenous system and perforator incompetence coexist where the perforating veins act as reentry veins allowing blood refluxing down the saphenous system to enter the deep veins. This may explain the observation by some[9,10] that perforator valve competence is restored after the saphenous system is removed.

Incompetent perforators often are seen associated with deep venous incompetence or obstruction. In this scenario, the perforators act as safety valves allowing blood under high pressure to escape and drive blood into the superficial veins causing enlargement of the capillaries and extravasation of intravascular contents into the interstitial space.

In the deep veins, primary valvular incompetence can be seen but in general is not as common as secondary venous disease. A study by Myers and colleagues[11] using duplex ultrasound revealed isolated deep venous reflux in only 8% of patients with C_5/C_6 CVI. Post-thrombotic damage within the deep veins is a more common cause of severe CVI (C_4–C_6) and usually involves a combination of reflux and obstruction. Residual thrombus is replaced by fibrous tissue that may cause either a complete obstruction or synechiae, which develops across the vein wall, obstructing the outflow or impeding valve function. Also, if thrombus is in direct contact with the valve cups and the vein is not fully recanalized as the thrombus organizes can lead to irreparable damage of the valve function with subsequent reflux.[12]

SKIN CHANGES AND VENOUS ULCERATIONS

The pathophysiological relationship between venous hypertension and ulceration remains unclear. Earlier hypotheses, such as that arteriovenous fistulae open in the dermis in response to venous hypertension, have been challenged by the use of positron emission tomography, which failed to confirm the presence of such fistulae.[13] Observations of a pericapillary fibrin cuff in the dermal capillary bed led to the speculation that interstitial fibrin might interfere with the passage of oxygen and other nutrients to the overlying skin.[14,15] However, recent theories dispute the idea that pure fibrin would act as a diffusion block.[16,17]

The findings of white cell depletion in the venous affluent of dependent limbs led to the theory of white cell trapping plugging the dermal capillaries. The subsequent sluggish capillary blood flow leads to hypoxia and neutrophil activation. The problem with this theory is that neutrophils have never been directly observed to obstruct capillary flow; however, there is evidence that leukocyte activation plays a role in the pathophysiology of CVI.

Current knowledge indicates that venous hypertension causes extravasation of macromolecules and red blood cells into the interstitium. Red blood cell degradation and interstitial proteins are potent chemoattractants responsible for the initial leukocyte recruitment.[7,18] This process remains controversial but macrophages and mast cells have been observed on electron microscopic examinations.[19] The presence of mast cells suggests a role in cytokine activation and tissue remodeling. Immunohistochemical analyses of dermal biopsies on patients with CVI have demonstrated the presence of transforming growth factor-β_1 (TGF-β_1), also vascular endothelial growth factor (VEGF) and platelet-derived growth factor (PDGF).[7] TGF-β_1 may cause tissue fibrosis by stimulating extracellular matrix production through effects on matrix metalloproteinases (MMPs). Extracellular matrix (ECM) deposition is controlled by MMPs and tissue inhibitors of matrix metalloproteinases (TIMPs) and TGF-β_1 is an inducer of TIMPs and inhibitor of MMP-1. In patients with advanced CVI, TGF-β_1 has been demonstrated in pathologic amounts and it is possible that the intense tissue fibrosis is caused by the excess of TGF-β_1.

CLINICAL ASSESSMENT AND DIAGNOSTIC EVALUATION OF ADVANCED CVI

During the initial interview, any history of previous thrombotic episodes, previous episodes of lower extremity cellulitis, leg ulcers, venous and nonvenous surgery of the lower extremities or pelvis, and arterial insufficiency symptoms and risk factors associated with it, such as diabetes mellitus, smoking, and hyperlipidemia should be noted.

Symptomatology includes leg aching, heaviness, venous claudication, and most patients with advanced CVI have some degree of edema.

Signs of CVI include corona phlebectatica (fan-shaped flare of small intradermal varices on the medial aspect of the ankle and foot) and skin changes, including lipodermatosclerosis, which in its chronic phase appears as shiny, hard, and pigmented skin. Venous ulcers are usually located in the malleoli and gaiter area, are more common in the medial aspect of the lower leg (70%), and about one-third of the time in the lateral aspect. They have irregular edges with neo-epithelialization and the base is pink and granulating but can also can be covered with yellow slough.

Physical examination should be performed with the patient in the standing position. First, inspect for signs of CVI, as previously mentioned. Palpate dilated varicose veins and also the area of lipodermatosclerosis to detect the extent of induration and tenderness. Perform an abdominal examination to rule out a mass that could be responsible for venous obstruction. Also, a pulse examination of the lower extremities, including femoral, popliteal, posterior tibial, and dorsal pedal pulses should be performed to exclude arterial insufficiency.

Duplex ultrasound has become the gold standard in the diagnosis of advanced CVI and has replaced the use of venous plethymosgraphs and continuous wave Dopplers. It is performed in the standing position and includes assessment of both reflux and obstruction in the deep, superficial, and perforating veins from the level of the inguinal ligament to the distal calf. Duplex ultrasonography distinguishes primary valvular reflux from the obstructive pattern of post-thrombotic disease and those veins with mix pattern of luminal scarring with an occlusive component and secondary reflux.

Venous reflux in the superficial and deep venous system by duplex is defined as reversal of flow that is greater than 0.5 second. Duplex criteria for diagnosing incompetent perforating veins (ICPVs) is based on size of the perforator at a fascia level of greater than 3.5 mm and presence with calf compression of reversal of flow from the deep to the superficial venous system.[20]

TREATMENT

General measures in the treatment of venous ulcers and advanced CVI is weight reduction, leg elevation, and walking exercise. Systemic factors that can affect wound healing should not be overlooked, such as immunosuppression, malnutrition, diabetes mellitus, arterial circulation, local infection, and congestive heart failure.

Compression therapy is the basic treatment modality in venous leg ulcers and has been validated in randomized trials,[21] but to be effective, compliance with treatment is essential. Before starting compression therapy, CVI must be established and severe arterial insufficiency of the ankle-brachial index (ABI) of less than 0.5 should be ruled out.

One form of compression therapy includes elastic stockings. Current guidelines suggest the use of below-the-knee stockings with a 30- to 40-mm Hg compression pressure to treat C_5–C_6 CVI.[22] Mayberry and colleagues[23] showed in a retrospective review that compliant patients healed their ulcers in 97% of cases with a recurrence of 29% at 5 years. Some of the advantages of stockings are the following: they are operator independent, unlike Unna's boot or multilayer bandages; stockings are also less bulky and perhaps more comfortable; and they can be worn with normal footwear and allow daily inspection of the wound, which is especially important for exudative wounds.

Unna's boot is a form of compression bandage requiring a 3- or 4-layer dressing. The bandage becomes stiff and nonstretched after drying, generating resting pressures up to 50 to 60 mm Hg in the distal lower leg; however, as is the case of most inelastic bandages, the initial resting pressure may drop about 25% several hours after placement owing to decrease of the volume of the leg.

Unna's boot is changed weekly. A disadvantage associated with it is that it has to be applied by trained personnel; therefore, it is operator dependant. Also, the ulcer cannot be monitored and the boot may be uncomfortable to wear, and in some patients it may cause contact dermatitis. In a 15-year review, Lippman and colleagues[24] showed a 73% venous ulcer healing in a median time of 9 weeks with Unna's boot dressings.

Multilayer compression elastic bandage dressings have certain advantages over nonstretch inelastic materials, such as more even distribution of compression, better absorption of wound exudates, and compression for longer periods of time. The pressure delivered depends on the number of layers applied, the elastic properties of the materials used, and the wrapping technique. The more layers of elastic bandages applied will increase the inelastic properties and stiffness (4-layer bandage, Profore system). These bandages should exert a pressure of about 40 mm Hg on the distal lower leg. In several randomized trials[25,26] comparing multilayer elastic bandages with short stretch bandages (inelastic systems), the 4-layer bandage system was associated with significantly shorter time to ulcer healing.

For patients unwilling or unable to use multilayer bandages or stockings because of arthritis or other medical conditions, Velcro-band gaiters, such as Circ-aid, are an alternative. The device consists of multiple adjustable compression bands that are held in place with Velcro. With the adjustable bands, the pressure of the device can be tailored to the size of the limb as edema decreases.

Intermittent pneumatic compression (IPC) can also be used in ulcer healing.[27] This is especially useful in patients unable to walk and in those with concomitant arterial insufficiency. ICP is able to reduce edema and enhance arterial blood flow.[28,29]

MEDICAL THERAPY FOR VENOUS LEG ULCERS

As for most wound healing, adequate nutrition is essential. Studies have shown an inadequate intake of proteins, vitamin C, and zinc in elderly patients with leg ulcers.[30] Consideration should be given to make sure that proteins and multivitamins are added to the diet of these patients.

For venous ulcers with active signs of infection such as cellulitis and septicemia, intravenous antibiotics are indicated. The use of topical antibiotics is more controversial. In a systemic analysis of randomized trials,[31] the use of topical antibiotics did not offer conclusive evidence of improved wound healing.

Prostaglandin E_1 (PGE-$_1$) has been evaluated in the treatment of venous ulcerations. In several trials,[32–34] intravenous PGE-$_1$ was shown to improve CVI symptoms, reduce edema, and increase rates of venous ulcer healing. However in one trial,[33] PGE-$_1$ was administered over 3 hours daily for 6 weeks. In another trial,[34] patients were treated for 20 days with PGE-$_1$ infusion. The long course of intravenous therapy is a clear disadvantage of this therapy.

Iloprost, a synthetic prostacyclin analog, has failed to show any significant benefit in healing of venous leg ulcers. In a study[35] where Iloprost was applied topically it showed no difference compared with placebo. Currently it has no role in the management if venous leg ulcers.

The only oral drugs that have shown to have a positive effect in healing of venous ulcers are pentoxifylline and micronized purified flavonoid fraction (MPFF). Both have been used in clinical trials as adjunctive therapy to compression and appropriate local wound care.

The use of pentoxifylline was validated in a recent review of 9 clinical trials,[36] which showed that pentoxifylline is an effective adjunct to compression therapy. Overall, there was an absolute increase in venous ulcer healing of 21% in those patients taking pentoxifylline plus compression compared with the placebo group.

Micronized purified flavonoid fraction (MPFF; Daflon 500), which consists of 90% Diosmin and 10% flavonoids, protects the microcirculation from damage secondary to increased ambulatory venous pressure.[37] In a recent meta-analysis,[38] MPFF used as an adjunctive to conventional therapy (compression + wound care) was compared with placebo plus conventional treatment. At 6 months, the chance of healing an ulcer was 32% higher in patients with adjunctive MPFF.

In the most recent treatment guidelines by the AVF,[39] the use of pentoxifylline or MPFF (in combination with compression) for large and chronic venous ulcers has a grade recommendation 1B.

SURGICAL TREATMENT OF ADVANCED CVI

Historically, with the exception of some isolated centers, surgeons in general have had a nihilistic approach to the surgical treatment of venous ulcers based on erroneous concepts, and the general belief in the futility of surgical therapy for advanced CVI.

However, recent evidence suggests a more important role for surgical management. First, the dogma that venous ulcers are caused only by deep venous disease has been disproved in recent years. Duplex studies have demonstrated that incompetence in the superficial venous system is common in patients with venous ulcers. In a study by Myers and colleagues,[11] isolated superficial reflux was seen in 39% of patients with CVI class 4 and 38% of patients with C_5 to C_6 disease. Combined superficial and deep reflux was observed in 48% of patients with venous ulcers. These results suggest that treatment directed to the superficial veins alone is helpful for a significant number of patients with advanced CVI.

Another concept that has been challenged is that treatment of superficial venous reflux in the presence of combined superficial and deep reflux is also futile. Studies have shown that especially in the presence of primary deep reflux and segmental deep venous reflux (DVR), elimination of superficial reflux may eliminate DVR. Puggioni and colleagues[40] showed that 30% of patients with primary axial DVR and 36% of patients with primary segmental DVR had resolution of DVR by duplex ultrasound after elimination of greater saphenous vein reflux. It is important to note that in this study, patients with prior history of DVT were excluded. Another study from the United Kingdom[41] examined the role of superficial venous surgery in patients with combined superficial venous reflux (SVR) and segmental DVR. Overall, duplex demonstrated postoperative resolution of segmental DVR in 49% of the limbs and ulcer healing occurred in 77% of limbs at 12 months.

The role of surgery has become more secure in the treatment of advanced CVI with the recent publication of randomized trials comparing surgery and compression with compression alone. Zanboni and colleagues[42] randomized 45 patients with venous leg ulcers and isolated SVR to compression alone (24 patients) and superficial venous surgery (21 patients) with the use of postoperative 20- to 30-mm Hg elastic stockings. The healing rate was 96% in a median period of 63 days for the compression group compared with 100% in a median of 31 days for the surgical group. Recurrence of venous ulcer was more common in the compression group (38%) versus the surgical group (9%).

The landmark study regarding the role of superficial venous surgery in advanced CVI is the ESCHAR study (Effect of Surgery and Compression on Healing And Recurrence in patients with chronic venous ulcers).[43] This study randomized 500 patients with advanced CVI (C_5–C_6). A total of 258 patients were allocated to compression alone and 242 to compression plus surgery. All patients had superficial venous incompetence demonstrated by duplex and normal ABI greater than 0.85. Patients with segmental and total or axial deep venous reflux were included in the study where 60% of patients had isolated superficial reflux, 25% had mixed superficial and segmental deep reflux, and 15% had mixed superficial and total or axial deep reflux.

Compression consisted of multilayer compression bandaging to achieve 40 mm Hg of pressure at the ankle. Surgery consisted of saphenofemoral or saphenopopliteal ligation, stripping of greater saphenous vein (GSV) to the knee or small saphenous veins, and varicosity avulsions. Deep venous reconstruction was not offered. Overall, 24-week healing rates were similar in the 2 groups (65% vs 65%), $P = .85$ but there was a major difference in recurrence rate with a 12-month ulcer recurrence rate of 28% for compression therapy alone versus only 12% for surgery plus compression. Subgroup analysis showed that even in patients with mixed superficial and segmental deep reflux, there was a lower ulcer recurrence rate of only 9% compared with 25% with compression alone ($P = .04$). No statistically significant difference in recurrence rates was seen in patients with total deep reflux (19% vs 31%) but still a tendency to lower recurrence in the surgical group. The investigators concluded that superficial venous surgery reduces venous ulcer recurrence and should be considered for all patients with venous ulceration.

SUPERFICIAL VENOUS SURGERY

Techniques for ablation of saphenous vein reflux include high ligation with stripping, endovenous thermal ablation, and foam sclerotherapy.

Saphenous vein stripping has been considered the gold standard for superficial venous surgery and most surgeons are familiar with this technique; however, over the past decade there has been an increase in the use of minimally invasive techniques for the treatment of greater and small saphenous vein reflux that have replaced traditional stripping in many practices in the United States today.

Radiofrequency ablation, also known as the closure procedure, was the first endovenous thermal ablation technique developed. The intervention delivers electromagnetic energy through a radiofrequency (RF) catheter and generator (VNUS Medical Technologies Inc, Sunnyvale, CA) to heat the vein wall and destroy the intima, resulting in fibrous occlusion of the vein. The procedure is performed under local anesthesia in an outpatient setting. The catheter is preferably introduced into the saphenous vein under ultrasound guidance and advanced up to the saphenofemoral (SF) junction and its position is confirmed by ultrasound. The catheter is usually placed distal to the epigastric tributary or 1 to 2 cm away from the SF junction. Local tumescent anesthetic is instilled in the subcutaneous tissues and surrounding the saphenous vein compartment to minimize pain, help to coat the vein walls around the catheter, and protect surrounding tissues. Graduated withdrawal of the catheter is performed and the heating is controlled by monitoring temperature and impedance of the vein wall.

Recently published 5-year data from the VNUS registry suggest that the closure procedure is effective. Vein occlusion at 1 year was documented by duplex ultrasound in 87.1% of the legs treated, 83.5% at 3 years, and 87.2% at 5 years.[44] The EVOLVES study[45] was a prospective randomized trial to compare the RF ablation procedure to the conventional ligation/stripping procedure with respect to short-term recovery and early results. This study revealed significant early advantages for the closure procedure with earlier recovery, overall less postoperative pain, earlier return to routine activities, and similar immediate early technical success.

Endovenous laser treatment of saphenous veins developed during the 1990s but received approval from the US Food and Drug administration in January 2002, and today is perhaps the most common method of saphenous ablation used in the United States.

Endovenous laser ablation (EVLA) delivers laser energy directly into the vein lumen causing the blood inside the vein to boil and the formation of steam bubbles induces local heat injury in the inner wall of the vein.[46] Heat transferred to the vein wall leads to shrinkage of vein wall collagen fibers and reduction of the lumen.

Laser generators are available from several manufacturers and different laser wave lengths of 810, 940, 1064, and 1320 mm are used but all different wave lengths have similar clinical results and the wave lengths seems not to be important for the success of EVLA.

The technique for EVLA is very similar to the one already described for the closure device also done with local anesthesia and in an outpatient setting. Laser energy is delivered by a stepwise or continuous fiber pullback. Depending on the manufacturer, the pullback is done manually or by use of monitored pullback devices, which is the case of the 1320-mm laser. Typical pullback speeds are in the range of 0.5 to 3.0 mm/s and the goal is to deliver a linear endovenous energy density (LEED) of approximately 80 J per cm vein length.[47]

Superior outcomes with this technique have been published. Min and colleagues[48] reported long-term follow-up results of 499 limbs treated with an 810-mm laser. Successful occlusion of the GSV by duplex was observed in 98.2% of limbs after initial treatment. At 2 years, 113 limbs were available for follow-up and 93.4% remained closed. Other investigators have reported occlusion rates of 95.2% at 12-month follow-up.[49]

Postoperative adverse events related to EVLA or VNUS closure include echymosis, pain, paresthesia, infection, cutaneous thermal injury, superficial thrombophlebitis, and deep vein thrombosis. The reported incidence of deep vein thrombus[50] is only about 1% to 2% and more often consists of thrombus extensions from the greater or small saphenous veins into the deep venous system (popliteal or common femoral vein). However, with careful Duplex follow-up most of these thrombus extensions retract over the course of 7 to 15 days and none produce clinical symptoms suggestive of pulmonary embolus.

By AVF clinical guidelines,[39] EVLA and VNUS closure of saphenous veins is regarded as safe and effective treatment of incompetence and has a grade 1A recommendation.

Another minimally invasive technique to achieve ablation of the saphenous vein is the use of foam sclerotherapy. Sclerosing foams are mixtures of gas with a liquid solution with surfactant properties such a sodium tetradecyl sulfate or polidocanol. Sclerosant agents cause endothelial damage with exposure of the subendothelial collagen leading to platelet aggregation with subsequent coagulation and endofibrosis of the vessel lumen.[51]

The sclerosing foam solution is injected into the saphenous veins under ultrasound guidance. As the foam reaches the SF junction or saphenopopliteal junction monitored by ultrasound, compression is applied to these junctions to reduce flowing foam into the deep system. Results of this therapy from Europe where the use of this technique is more widespread than in the United States are available. A prospective multicenter study conducted in France showed absence of GSV reflux at 1 month after foam sclerotherapy.[52]

There are also data using sclerosant foam for superficial vein ablation in patients with CEAP 4, 5, and 6 limbs. Pascarella and colleagues[53] compared foam sclerotherapy with compression alone in advanced CVI. They found better efficacy with foam sclerotherapy versus compression alone in ulcer healing (70% vs 50%, respectively).

PERFORATORS

Much debate exists in the literature and among various specialists regarding the hemodynamic significance and clinical significance of perforating veins in the development of advanced CVI (C_4–C_6).

The hemodynamic significance is difficult to determine because isolated perforator incompetence in advanced CVI is present in fewer than 5% of patients and most patients display concomitant superficial or deep venous incompetence.

In patients with advanced CVI, duplex studies have shown a significant prevalence of incompetent perforators. The Edinburgh group showed that the deteriorating CEA grade of CVI was associated with an increase in the number and diameter of medial calf perforating veins with the presence of 6% incompetent perforators for patients with $CEAP_0$ versus 90% in patients with $CEAP_{5-6}$.[54]

Despite these anatomic findings, the relative clinical significance of the perforator veins is still a matter of debate. The question that remains is whether they independently contribute to severe CVI or they are just a secondary effect of superficial or deep venous incompetence.

Mendes and colleagues[55] studied patients with concomitant saphenous reflux and incompetent perforators (IPVs) but without DVI with duplex and functional studies including air plethysmography (APG). A total of 24 patients underwent saphenous vein stripping and phlebectomies. Postoperative duplex scan demonstrated that 71% of previous IVPs were competent or absent and significant improvement in all APG values were documented. Other investigators[10] have shown that although there is a decrease in the number of IPVs after complete ablation of the GSV (52% preoperatively vs 28% postoperatively), in those patients with concomitant DVI, saphenous surgery alone fails to connect IPV reflux, showing 72% of limbs with persistent IPVs after superficial reflux ablation.

INDICATIONS AND TECHNIQUES FOR PERFORATOR VEIN INTERRUPTION

Although still controversial, many investigators consider a potential indication the presence of IPVs in patients with advanced CVI (C_4–C_6), including those with isolated IPVs as well as those combined with superficial or deep venous incompetence. In the group of superficial venous plus IPV incompetence, combined superficial and perforator vein reflux ablation is a reasonable approach; however, the procedures also could be staged reserving perforator interruption after saphenous ablation only for those patients with persistent problems.

Elimination of perforator reflux can be performed using a variety of techniques. Open surgical ligation, mini-incision ligation, subfascial endoscopic ligation, and percutaneous ablation with sclerosant foam or thermal energy can all be considered.

No randomized prospective trials exist comparing the effectiveness of these techniques.

Open surgeries such as the original Linton procedure carried a high incidence of wound complications.[56,57] For this reason, alternate methods were developed to eliminate the need for surgical incisions. The most widely performed is endoscopic or laparoscopic subfascial perforator ligation (SEPS). Two main techniques for SEPS have been developed. The single-port technique uses mediastinoscopes and bronchoscopes and the more recent and widely used "2-port" technique uses standard laparoscopic instrumentation and the use of carbon dioxide insufflation into the subfascial plane. All perforators encountered are divided with harmonic scalpel, electrocautery, or clips. Also, a pretibial fasciotomy is made by opening the fascia of the posterior deep compartment allowing visualization of proximal paratibial perforator veins. However, retromalleolar Cockett I perforators usually cannot be reached endoscopically.

With the advent of SEPS, the wound complication rates of perforator vein ablation and prolonged recovery were not a major concern, and this technique was embraced by many surgeons in both Europe and North America. Despite reports documenting safety, rapid ulcer healing, and early low recurrence rate with SEPS, controversy still exists in how much clinical improvement can be attributed to SEPS alone, as two-thirds of patients in these series also had concomitant saphenous vein stripping and varicose vein avulsion.

Gloviczki and colleagues[58] reported the midterm results from the North American Subfascial Endoscopic Perforator Surgery Registry. A total of 146 patients underwent SEPS; 69% had active ulcers and 14% had healed ulcers. Also, 71% of patients underwent concomitant superficial venous procedures. Cumulative ulcer healing at 1 year was 88% but cumulative ulcer recurrence at 1 year was 16% and at 2 years was 28%. Their wound complication rate was only 6% and they noted their worst overall results with patients with secondary CVI and mixed DVI with persistent deep venous occlusion and incompetence. In this group, ulcer recurrence rate was 46%. However, SEPS resulted in a significant clinical improvement in patients with non-thrombotic CVI.

Tenbrook and colleagues[59] did a systemic review of 20 reported series of SEPS involving 1140 limbs. In these series, 88% of ulcers healed and their recurrence was only 13% at a mean time of 21 months. They identified risk factors for nonhealing and recurrence included persistent IPVs, deep venous obstruction, and ulcer larger than 2 cm.

Others have reported even more encouraging results. Tawes and colleagues[60] in a multicenter, retrospective review of 832 patients who underwent SEPS for CVI (C_4–C_6), ulcer healing was achieved or significantly improved in 92% of patients in a mean of 7 weeks and ulcer recurrence was only 4%. In this study, 55% of patients underwent concomitant saphenous vein ligation and stripping and 28% of patients had DVI.

One randomized trial, the Dutch SEPS trial[61] comparing medical treatment (compression) versus SEPS (with or without superficial ablation) showed a similar recurrence rate at 29 months of 22% for the surgical arm versus 23% for the medical therapy. In a follow-up study,[62] the same group reported that the ulcer-free rate was significantly greater in the surgical group (72% vs 53%).

The AVF guidelines[39] regarding the management of IPVs in patients with advanced venous disease with endoscopic surgery have a 2B grade recommendation.

A more novel modality of therapy is percutaneous ablation of perforating veins (PAPs) with either chemical or thermal energy. Theoretical advantages over SEPS include the use of only local anesthesia for this procedure and it is also office-based.

There is no need for dissection and the location of perforating veins does not matter with PAPs. Even perforators close to the malleolus are easily accessible. PAPs is also easily repeatable with minimal morbidity. Disadvantages include missed IPVs by ultrasound and the need of being quite familiar with ultrasound-guided percutaneous access.

The technique is relatively simple. First, ultrasound-guided access to the perforator with either a 21-gauge micropuncture needle, angio catheter, or a 25-gauge needle depending on the type of ablation used. Once access is obtained, it is important to stay at the fascia or above it to minimize risk of DVT or nerve injury. Next, some form of ablative energy (chemical or thermal) is used within the perforators and finally confirmation of initial treatment success is performed with ultrasound.

Chemical ablation is performed with sclerosants such as sodium tetradecyl sulfate (sotradecol) or Polidocanol. To obtain a greater sclerosing ability, the liquid sclerosant is mixed with gas (air or CO2) to obtain microfoam sclerotherapy.[63] Cabrera and colleagues[64] followed 116 patients with venous ulcers and IPVs treated with ultrasound-guided injection of polidocanol foam. At 6 months, 86% of patients achieved complete healing. They observed that presence of deep venous incompetence and chronicity of the ulcer were independent risk factors of failure to achieve complete healing. At 24 months, the overall recurrence rate was 6.3%. Thermal ablation can be performed with either radiofrequency catheter or laser energy. Chang and colleagues[65] reported a 12-month follow-up posttreatment of 38 IPVs with radiofrequency ablation. At 1 year, 91% were reflux free; however, 56% were patent, which reveals that posttreatment patency not always translates into incompetence. Longer follow-up will be needed to show any meaningful conclusions.

Kabnick[66] presented data on 25 IPVs treated with laser energy that showed 85% closure rate at 4 months. Elias[67] showed a 90% occlusion at 1 month of 50 IPVs treated with laser energy (810 mm wave length). Proebstle and Herdemanns[68] showed a 99% occlusion rate in 67 IPVs at 3-month follow-up. PAPs is rapidly growing in popularity among venous surgeons because of its minimal invasiveness and because it is a procedure that is easily repeatable if necessary. Further studies with longer follow-up will be needed to validate this procedure in the treatment of patients with advanced CVI.

By current AVF guidelines,[39] PAPs has a recommendation of 2C for the treatment of IPVs given the still low-quality scientific data. We suspect that this will change in the future as more data will become available.

SIGNIFICANCE OF CHRONIC PROXIMAL VENOUS OUTFLOW OBSTRUCTION

For many years, the clinical practice of advanced CVI has evolved around venous reflux while venous obstruction largely has been ignored. With the development of minimally invasive techniques to treat ileo-caval pathology and the use of intravascular ultrasound (IVUS) as a new diagnostic tool[69,70] to better define the anatomy and intrinsic or extrinsic compression lesions of major outflow veins, there has been an increased interest to understand the role that proximal venous outflow obstruction may play in the pathogenesis of advanced CVI.

Obstructive pathology or major outflow veins can be attributable to thrombotic obstruction after poor recanalization following acute deep vein thrombosis. It has been shown that only about 20% of iliac veins after DVI will completely recanalize on anticoagulation treatment. The remaining will develop varying degrees of obstruction and collateral formation.[71,72] Venous claudication has been found in 15% to 44%

and venous ulcers have developed in up to 15% of patients because of post thrombotic iliac venous disease.[71,73]

Another form of obstructive pathology is nonthrombotic, nonmalignant primary obstruction (NIVL). May-Thurner Syndrome Type:[74] left proximal common iliac vein stenosis caused by right iliac artery compression has been well described; however, it is not isolated to young women and compression lesions are not uncommon in males and elderly patients and may involve the right iliac veins.[75] Also, outflow obstruction can be related to the presence of intraluminal lesions. Ehrich and Krumbhar[76] described a high prevalence of obstructive intraluminal lesions in iliac veins (30% in 412 unselected autopsies).

The prevalence of these primary nonthrombotic iliac vein lesions is perhaps higher than originally thought. In a recent retrospective review, Neglen and Raju[75] reported that among 938 limbs with iliac vein obstructive lesions that 53% of the limbs had NIVL, 40% were post-thrombotic, and 7% a combination. Despite these anatomic findings, still there is lack of an accurate objective noninvasive or invasive test for evaluation of hemodynamically significant chronic venous obstruction. Ultrasound investigation and plethysmographic studies have been shown to be unreliable, and significant blockage may exist in the presence of normal findings.[77] Because hemodynamic tests are unreliable, diagnosis has been based on anatomic and morphologic findings. Noninvasive tests, such as CT and magnetic resonance venogram have been used successfully for acute ileofemoral DVT and obstructions of large veins in chest, abdomen, and pelvis. However, their role in workup of more subtle venous stenosis is not yet defined. Venogram has been the gold standard test. However, it may underestimate the degree of stenosis by 30%, especially in the anterior-posterior view. Increased accuracy may be achieved with multiple angle projections.[78] Intravascular ultrasound (IVUS) has shown to be superior to simple plain venography to detect the extent and degree of venous stenosis.[70,79,80] IVUS shows intraluminal details such as webs, reveals external compression and wall thickness, and is becoming the best available method for diagnosing clinically significant chronic iliac vein obstruction.

Patients with proximal venous outflow obstruction with disabling symptoms or advanced CVI (C_4–C_6) that failed medical management with compression and lifestyle modifications should be considered for venous reconstructions. Endovascular repair should be considered the first line of therapy given its relative simplicity, efficacy, and safety compared with open surgery. Venous stenting has been used to successfully treat iliac vein obstruction. Hartung and colleagues[81] reported their experience with 44 patients with ileocaval stenosis or occlusion. The etiology was primary in 73% of patients and secondary (post thrombotic) in 23%. Other etiologies such as hypoplasia or retroperitoneal fibrosis were present in 7%. Technical success of stenting was 95.5%. Median follow-up was 27 months. Cumulative primary, assisted primary, and secondary patency were 73%, 88%, and 90% respectively.

The clinical impact of correcting outflow venous problems with iliac venous stents in patients with advanced CVI has been reported. Raju and colleagues[82] published their experience with 304 limbs with symptomatic CVI. Of those, 122 patients had C_4–C_6 and 158 patients had leg edema (C_3). There were a total of 49 patients with venous ulcers. Associated reflux was present in 57% of the limbs. In median follow-up of 7 months (range 2 to 35), 68% of venous ulcers healed, 16% improved, and only 4% recurred. Notably there was no difference in ulcer healing after stent placement alone as compared in a subgroup with stent and correction of superficial reflux. The same group has published their 5-year data with respect to iliac vein stent patency, which has been a concern of many practitioners. Raju and colleagues reported a cumulative primary and assisted primary patency rate of 75% and 94% respectively.[83]

In the AVF's most recent guidelines,[39] endovenous stenting for chronic iliac vein obstruction to improve symptoms and quality of life of patients with CVD has a grade IA recommendation.

Open surgical reconstruction for patients with venous obstructive disease of the ileofemoral veins or IVC should be reserved for those patients with advanced CVI who are not candidates or after failed attempts at endovascular reconstruction.

Patients with unilateral iliac vein obstruction are candidates for a femoro-femoral crossover bypass (Palma procedure). The greater saphenous vein should be the conduit of preference but for those patients without a GSV or inadequate size vein (<3 or 4 mm) a 10 mm, externally supported PTFE graft can be used. Jost and colleagues[84] reported their experience with 18 saphenous vein crossover grafts. Four-year primary and secondary patency rates were 77% and 83% respectively. Halliday and colleagues[85] reported 47 Palma procedures with saphenous vein with 75% patency rate at 60-month follow-up. Overall cumulative patency of prosthetic femoro-femoral bypass is somewhat lower (60%–67%).[86,87]

For patients with bilateral iliac, ileocaval, or IVC occlusion, a femoro-ilio-caval bypass is another surgical option. These venous reconstructions are performed with ePTFE graft or with spiral vein grafts. According to the anatomy of the venous obstructions, several reconstructions are possible, including femorocaval, ileocaval, or cavoatrial. For long PTFE grafts (>10 cm) to improve their patency, many investigators recommend an adjunctive arteriovenous fistula[88,89] at the groin level. Only a few centers have significant experience with these more complex venous reconstructions. The Mayo group reported their experience in 14 patients with ileocaval and femorocaval bypasses (femorocaval 8, ileocaval 5, cavoatrial 1, all with PTFE graft) and 6 patients with spiral vein grafts (5 iliac/femoral and 1 cavoatrial). At 2 years, the primary patency and secondary patency for ileo and femorocaval bypass with PTFE was 38% and 54% respectively. Four (67%) of 6 spiral grafts were patent.[84] Sottiurai[90] noted slight better results with 16 of 19 ePTFE grafts being patent during follow-up of 80 to 113 months following femorocaval and femoroiliac bypasses. Also, ulcer healing was noted in 10 (77%) of 13 of patients.

Regarding open surgical reconstructions, the AVF guidelines[39] have a grade IB recommendation for a cross pubic bypass (Palma procedure) with saphenous vein for symptomatic patients with unilateral ileofemoral venous occlusion after failed attempts of endovascular reconstructions.

For symptomatic patients with iliac vein or IVC occlusion, reconstruction with open bypass with externally supported PTFE graft has a grade 2B recommendation.

SURGICAL REPAIR OF DEEP VEIN VALVE INCOMPETENCE

Deep valve repair is a well established surgical procedure first described by Dr Kistner.[91] However, despite several series reporting up to 65% to 80% healing of venous ulcers,[92,93] these procedures have remained the niche of only a small group of surgeons around the country.

Deep venous valve surgical repair should be considered only in those patients with advanced CVI (class 3 or higher) with disabling symptoms such as severe venous claudication, recurrent nonhealing venous ulcers, recurrent cellulitis in patients with edema and advanced venous stasis changes who have exhausted other less invasive therapeutic options such as compression therapy, ablation of refluxive saphenous veins, or perforators and once proximal outflow venous obstruction whether post thrombotic or NIVL has been ruled out and first corrected through stent placement.

Patients considered for surgery should undergo a detail venous evaluation including duplex ultrasound, air plethysmography, and ascending and descending venograms.

There are multiple surgical techniques to address valve incompetence and the choice of the technique will depend on if one is addressing "primary valve reflux or post-thrombotic disease" but more importantly, the best technique will be decided intraoperatively depending on whether the valve section appears normal or whether there is damage to the valve with perivenous and wall fibrosis sometimes rendering the valve nonrepairable. Specific valve reconstruction techniques are beyond the scope of this article, but in general there are direct valve repair techniques including internal valvuloplasty and its different modifications,[89,92] external valvuloplasty,[94] angioscopic repair,[95] transcommissural valvuloplasty,[96] and prosthetic sleeve.[97] These direct techniques should be used first if the valve structure is repairable and in general are used more frequently in primary valve reflux.

There are also indirect techniques, such as segment transfer,[98] axillary vein transfer,[92,99,100] and neovalves.[101,102] They should be used only if direct repair fails or is not feasible.

Several controversies exist about valve reconstructions regarding the preferred site for valve repair, whether it is the femoral valve or the popliteal valve and whether a single valve repair is enough or whether multiple valve repairs would yield better results. Also valve reconstruction in post-thrombotic veins is controversial because of poorer results in some series compared with repair in primary valve reflux.[92,93] Raju and colleagues[103] reported one of the largest experiences with a total of 423 valve repairs in 258 limbs with a follow-up period that ranged from 1 to 12 years. Venous reflux was considered primary in 62% and post thrombotic in 38% of patients. Different surgical techniques were used and in 128 limbs a single valve was reconstructed versus 130 limbs where multiple valves were repaired. Of the 258 limbs, 211 (82%) were operated for ulcerations. Of these, about 4.7% never healed and about 20.3% recurred during the observation period. Another observation was that ulcer recurrence was not different among the various surgical techniques or between single and multiple valve repairs. The site of valve repair showed a significant advantage for proximal superficial femoral vein compared with all other locations.

Kistner also published long-term results of venous valve reconstruction in 51 extremities with advanced CVI and a minimum follow-up period of 4 years (range 4 to 21 years). Kistner used different surgical procedures, including femoral valve repair (internal valvuloplasty), transposition, and transplantation (axillary vein transfer). He reported a 10-year cumulative success rate of 73% for patients with primary venous insufficiency and only 43% for patients with post thrombotic syndrome.[93]

By the AVF's most recent guidelines,[39] valve reconstruction in primary valvular incompetence after less invasive therapies had failed, and has a grade 1A recommendation and after post-thrombotic cases has a 2B recommendation.

SUMMARY

Venous ulcers are chronic, often recurrent, and very disabling conditions for many unfortunate patients who suffer this disease, often for many years. Surgeons in general and other physicians that care for these patients should abandon the nihilistic approach in the treatment of venous ulcers. The focus should be on the venous disorder causing the ulcer. An aggressive diagnostic workup and identification of the venous pathology should be established, and medical and step-fashion surgical treatment should be tailored accordingly.

REFERENCES

1. Callam MJ. Epidemiology of varicose veins. Br J Surg 1994;81:167–73.
2. Rabe E, Pannier-Fisher F, Bromen K, et al. Bonner Venenstudie der Deutschen Gesellschaft fur Phlebologic—epidemiologigische Untersuchung zur Frage der Haufigkeit und Avspragung von chronischen Venenkrakheiten inder stadtischen un landlichen wohnbevolkerung. Phlebologic 2003;32:1–14 [in German].
3. Jawien D, Gorzela T, Ochwat D. Prevalence of chronic venous insufficiency in men and women in Poland: multicenter cross-sectional study in 40,085 patients. Phlebology 2003;18:110–21.
4. Heit JA, Rooke TW, Silverstein MD, et al. Trends in the incidence of venous stasis syndrome and venous ulcer: a 25 year population-based study. J Vasc Surg 2001;33:1022–7.
5. Porter JM, Moneta GL. Reporting standards in venous disease: an update. International Consensus Committee in Chronic Venous Disease. J Vasc Surg 1995; 21:635–45.
6. Thomas PR, Nash GB, Dormandy JA. White cell accumulation in dependent legs of patients with venous hypertension: a possible mechanism for trophic changes in the skin. Br Med J (Clin Res Ed) 1988;296:1693–5.
7. Hisley HR, Ksander GA, Gerhardt CO, et al. Extravasation of macromolecules and possible trapping of transforming growth factor beta in venous ulceration. Br J Dematol 1995;132:79–85.
8. Alexander CJ. The theoretical basis of varicose vein formation. Med J Aust 1972;1:258–61.
9. Campbell WA, West A. Duplex ultrasound of operative treatment of varicose veins. In: Negus P, Jantet C, Smith P, editors. Phlebology. Berlin: Springer; 1995.
10. Stuart WP, Allan PL, Ruckley CV, et al. Saphenous surgery does not correct perforator incompetence in the presence of deep venous reflux. J Vasc Surg 1998;28:834–8.
11. Myers KA, Ziegenbein RW, Zeng GH, et al. Duplex ultrasonography scanning for chronic venous disease: patterns of venous reflux. J Vasc Surg 1995;21:605–12.
12. Edward EA, Edwards JE. The effect of thrombophlebitis on the venous valves. Surg Gynecol Obstet 1937;65:310–20.
13. Hopkins NF, Spinks TJ, Rhodes CG, et al. Positron emission tomography in venous ulceration and liposclerosis: a study of regional tissue formation. Br Med J 1983;6:9–14.
14. Burnand KG, Whimster I, Naidoo A, et al. Pericapillary fibrin in the ulcer bearing skin of the leg. Br Med J 1982;2:243–5.
15. Browse NL, Burnand KG. The cause of venous ulceration. Lancet 1982;2:243–5.
16. Michel CC. Aetiology of venous ulceration. Br J Surg 1990;77:1071.
17. Van De Scheur M, Falanga V. Pericapillary fibrin cuffs in venous disease. Dermatol Surg 1997;23:955–99.
18. Herrkk SE, Sloan P, McGuire M, et al. Sequential changes in histologic pattern and extracellular matrix deposition during the healing of chronic venous ulcers. Am J Pathol 1992;141:1085–95.
19. Pappas PJ, DeFouw DO, Venezio LM, et al. Morphometric assessment of the dermal microcirculation in patients with chronic venous insufficiency. J Vasc Surg 1997;26:784–95.

20. Delis KT, Husmann M, Kalodiki E, et al. In situ hemodynamics of perforating veins in chronic venous insufficiency. J Vasc Surg 2001;33(4):773–82.
21. Cullum M, Nelson ED, Fletcher DW, et al. Compression for venous leg ulcers. Cochrane Database Syst Rev 2001;2:CD 000265.
22. Partsch H. Evidence-based compression therapy. VASA 2003;32(Suppl 63):36.
23. Mayberry JC, Moneta GL, Taylor LM Jr, et al. Fifteen year results of ambulatory compression therapy for chronic venous ulcers. Surgery 1991;109:575.
24. Lippmann HI, Fishman LM, Farrar RH, et al. Edema control in the management of disabling chronic venous insufficiency. Arch Phys Med Rehabil 1994;75:436.
25. O'Meara S, Tierney J, Cullum M, et al. Four layer bandage compared with short stretch bandage for venous leg ulcer: systemic review and meta-analysis of randomized controlled trials with data from individual patients. BMJ 2009;338: B1344.
26. Ukat A, Konig M, Vanscheit W, et al. Short-stretch versus multilayer compression for venous leg ulcers: a comparison of healing rates. J Wound Care 2003; 12(No 4):139–43.
27. Mani R, Vowden K, Nelson EA. Intermittent pneumatic compression for treating venous leg ulcers. Cochrane Database Syst Rev 2001;23:CD001899.
28. Delis KT, Nicolaides DM, Wolfe JH. Improving walking ability and ankle brachial pressure indices in symptomatic peripheral vascular disease using intermittent pneumatic foot compression: a prospective controlled study with one year follow-up. J Vasc Surg 2000;31:650–61.
29. Eze AR, Comerota AJ, Cisek PL, et al. Intermittent calf and foot compression increases lower extremity blood flow. Am J Surg 1996;172:130–4.
30. Wipke-Tevis DD, Scotts NA. Nutrition, tissue oxygenation and healing of venous leg ulcers. J Vasc Nurs 1998;16:48–56.
31. O'Meara SM, Cullum NA, Majid M, et al. Systemic review of antimicrobial agents used for chronic wounds. Br J Surg 2001;88:4–21.
32. Beitner J, Hamar J, Olsson AG. Prostaglandin E_1 treatment of leg ulcers caused by venous or arterial incompetence. Acta Derm Venereol 1980;60:425–30.
33. Rudosfsky G. Intravenous prostaglandin E_1 in the treatment of venous ulcers: a double-blind, placebo controlled trial. VASA 1989;28(Suppl):39–43.
34. Milio G, Mina C, Caspite V, et al. Efficacy of the treatment with prostaglandin E_1 in venous ulcers of the lower limbs. J Vasc Surg 2005;42:304–8.
35. Werner-Schlenzka H, Kuhlmann RK. Treatment of venous leg ulcers with topical Iloprost: a placebo controlled study. VASA 1994;23:145–50.
36. Jull AB, Waters J, Droll B. Pentoxifylline for treating venous leg ulcers. Cochrane Database Syst Rev 2002;1:CD001733.
37. Lyseng-Williamson KA, Penny CM. Micronised purified flavonoid fraction. A review of its use in chronic venous insufficiency, venous ulcers and haemorrhoids. Drugs 2003;63:71–100.
38. Coleridge-Smith P, Lok C, Ramelet AA. Venous leg ulcer: a meta-analysis of adjunctive therapy with micronized purified flavonoid fraction. Eur J Vasc Endovasc Surg 2005;30:198–208.
39. Gloviczki P. Handbook of venous disorders. 3rd edition. Guidelines of the American venous forum, 2009.
40. Puggioni P, Kistner RL, Eklof BO. How often is deep venous reflux eliminated after saphenous vein ablation? J Vasc Surg 2003;38:517–21.
41. Adam DJ, Bello M, Hartshornet T, et al. Role of superficial venous surgery in patients with combined superficial and segmental deep venous reflux. Eur J Vasc Endovasc Surg 2003;25:469–72.

42. Zanboni P, Cisno C, Mazza P, et al. Minimally invasive surgical management of primary venous ulcers vs. compression treatment: a randomized clinical trial. Eur J Vasc Endovasc Surg 2003;25:313–8.

43. Barwell JR, Deacon J, Harvery K, et al. Comparison of surgery and compression with compression alone in chronic venous ulceration (Eschar Study): randomized controlled trial. Lancet 2004;363:1854–9.

44. Merchant RF, Pichot O. Long term outcomes of endovenous radio frequency obliteration of saphenous reflux as a treatment for superficial venous insufficiency. J Vasc Surg 2005;42(3):502–9.

45. Lurie F, Creton D, Eklof B, et al. Prospective randomized study of endovenous radio frequency obliteration (closure procedure) venous ligation and stripping in a selected patient population (Evolves study). J Vasc Surg 2003;38:207–14.

46. Proebstle TM, Lehr HA, Kagl A, et al. Endovenous treatment of the greater saphenous vein with a 940 mm duole laser. Thrombotic occlusion after endoluminal thermal damage by laser generated steam bubbles. J Vasc Surg 2002;35:729–36.

47. Proebstle TM. Energy delivery and pullback rates during EVL: how one does decide? Miami (FL): International Vein Congress; 2005.

48. Min RJ, Khilnani M, Zimmet E. Endovenous laser treatment of saphenous vein reflux: long term results. J Vasc Interv Radiol 2003;14:991–6.

49. Bone C, Navarro L. Endovenous laser: a new minimally invasive technique for the treatment of varicose veins. Ann Cir Cardiaca Cir Vasc 2001;29:357–61.

50. Mozes G, Kalra M, Carmo M, et al. Extension of saphenous thrombus into the femoral vein: a potential complication of new endovenous techniques. J Vasc Surg 2005;41:130–5.

51. Bergan IJ. Excision of varicose veins. In: Eernst CB, Stanley JC, editors. Current therapy in vascular surgery. 4th edition. St Louis (MO): Mosby; 2001. p. 838–40.

52. Cabrera J, Cabrera J Jr, Garcia-Almeida A. Treatment of varicose long saphenous veins with sclerosant in microfoam form: long term outcomes. Phlebology 2000;15:19–23.

53. Pascarella L, Bergan JJ, Mckenas LV. Severe chronic venous insufficiency treated by foamed sclerosant. Ann Vasc Surg 2006;20:83–91.

54. Stuart WP, Adam PJ, Allan PL, et al. The relationship between the number, competence, and diameter of medial calf perforating veins and the clinical status in healthy subjects and patients with lower-limb venous disease. J Vasc Surg 2000;32:138–43.

55. Mendes RR, Manston WA, Faber MA, et al. Treatment of superficial and perforator venous incompetence without deep venous insufficiency: is routine perforator ligation necessary? J Vasc Surg 2003;38:891–5.

56. Linton RR. The communicating veins of the lower leg and the operative technique for their ligation. Ann Surg 1938;107:582.

57. Stuart VP, Asain DJ, Ruckley CV. Subfascial endoscopic perforator surgery is associated with significantly less morbidity and shorter hospital stay than open operation. Br J Surg 1997;84:1364–5.

58. Gloviczki P, Bergan JJ, Rhodes JM, et al. Midterm results of endoscopic perforator vein interruption for chronic venous insufficiency: lessons learned from North American subfascial endoscopic perforator surgery registry. J Vasc Surg 1999;29:489–502.

59. Tenbrook JA, Iafrati MD, O'Donnel TF, et al. Systemic review of outcomes after surgical management of venous disease incorporating subfascial endoscopic perforator surgery. J Vasc Surg 2004;39:583–9.

60. Tawes RL, Barron ML, Coello AA, et al. Optimal therapy for advanced chronic venous insufficiency. J Vasc Surg 2003;37:545–51.

61. Wittens CH, Van Gent BW, Hop WC, et al. The patch subfascial endoscopic perforating vein surgery (SEPS) trial: a randomized multicenter trial comparing ambulatory compression therapy versus surgery in patients with venous leg ulcers. Chicago: Society for Vascular Surgery; 2003.

62. Van Gent WB, Hop WC, Van Praag MC. Conservative versus surgical treatment of venous leg ulcers: a prospective, randomized, multicenter trial. Perspect Vasc Surg Endovasc Ther 2006;18:347–9.

63. Cabrera J, Redondo P. Foam treatment of venous leg ulcers: the initial experience. In: Bergan JJ, Shortell CK, editors. Venous ulcers. Copyright Elsevier Inc; 2007. p. 199–213.

64. Cabrera J, Redondo P, Becerra A, et al. Ultrasound guided injection of polidocanal microfoam in the management of venous leg ulcers. Arch Dermatol 2004; 140:667–73.

65. Chang DW, Levy D, Hayashi RM, et al. Ultrasound-guided radiofrequency ablation (VNUS) can be used to treat perforator incompetence: 1 year results and how to do it. Vascular 2005;13:518.

66. Kabnick L. Perforator vein treatment. In: Presented at the vein meeting, Uncasville (CT), 2006.

67. Elias S. PAPS: a minimally invasive treatment for incompetent perforating veins. In: Presented at the society for clinical vascular surgery annual meeting, scientific session, 2007.

68. Proebstle TM, Herdemann S. Early results and feasibility of incompetent perforator vein ablation by endovenous laser treatment. Dermatol Surg 2007;33: 162–8.

69. Ahmed HK, Hagspiel KD. Intravascular ultrasonographic findings in May-Thurner Syndrome (Iliac vein compression syndrome). J Ultrasound Med 2001;20:251–6.

70. Neglén P, Raju S. Intravascular ultrasound scan evaluation of the obstructed vein. J Vasc Surg 2002;35:694–700.

71. Akesson H, Buedin L, Eklof B, et al. Venous function assessed during a 5 year period after acute ileofemoral venous thrombosis treated with anticoagulants. Eur J Vasc Surg 1990;4:43–8.

72. Plate G, Akesson H, Einarsson E, et al. Long term results of venous thrombectomy combined with a temporary arterio-venous fistula. Eur J Vasc Surg 1990;4: 483–9.

73. Delis KT, Mansfield AO. Venous claudication in ileofemoral thrombosis: long term effects on venous hemodynamics, clinical status, and quality of life. Ann Surg 2004;239:118–26.

74. May R, Thurner J. The cause of the predominantly sinistral occurrence of the thrombosis of the pelvic veins. Angiology 1957;8:419–27.

75. Raju S, Neglen P. High prevalence of non thrombotic iliac vein lesions in chronic venous disease: a permissive role in pathogenicity. J Vasc Surg 2006;44: 136–44.

76. Ehrich WE, Krumbhaar EB. A frequent obstructive anomaly of the mouth of the left common iliac vein. Ann Heart J 1943;26:737–50.

77. Labropoulos M, Volteas M, Leon M, et al. The role of venous outflow obstruction in patients with chronic venous dysfunction. Arch Surg 1997;132:46–51.

78. Juhan C, Alimini Y, Harting O, et al. Treatment of non malignant obstructive ileocaval lesions by stent placement: mid term results. Ann Vasc Surg 2001;15: 227–32.

79. Fonaver AR, Gemmete JJ, Dasika NL, et al. Intravascular ultrasound in the diagnosis and treatment of iliac vein compression (May Thurner) Syndrome. J Vasc Interv Radiol 2002;13:523-7.
80. Satokawa H, Hoshino S, Igari I, et al. Intravascular image methods for venous disorders. Int Angiol 2000;9:117-21.
81. Hartung O, Otero O, Borfi M, et al. Mid term results of endovascular treatment for symptomatic chronic non malignant ileocaval venous occlusive disease. J Vasc Surg 2005;42:1138-44.
82. Raju S, Owen S, Meglen P. The clinical impact of iliac venous stents in the management of chronic venous insufficiency. J Vasc Surg 2002;35:8-15.
83. Peter N. Treatment of iliac venous obstruction in chronic venous disease. In: Bergan JJ, editor. The vein book. Elsevier Inc; 2007. p. 549-57.
84. Jost CT, Gloviczki P, Cherry KJ, et al. Surgical reconstruction of ileofemoral veins and the inferior vena cava for non malignant occlusive disease. J Vasc Surg 2001;33:320-8.
85. Halliday P, Harris J, May J. Femoro-femoral crossover grafts (Palma operation): a long term follow up study. Surgery of the veins. Orlando (FL): Grune & Stratton; 1985. p. 241-54.
86. Yamamoto M. Reconstruction with insertion of expanded polytetrafluorethylene (PTFE) graft for iliac venous obstruction. J Cardiovasc Surg 1986;27:697-702.
87. Comerota AJ, Aldridge SC, Cohen G, et al. A strategy of aggressive regional therapy for acute ileofemoral thrombosis with contemporary venous thrombectomy or catheter directed thrombolysis. J Vasc Surg 1994;20:244-54.
88. Menawat SS, Gloviczki P, Mozes G, et al. Effect of a femoral arteriovenous fistula on lower extremity venous hemodynamics after femorocaval reconstruction. J Vasc Surg 1996;24:793-9.
89. Eklof B. The temporary arteriovenous fistula in venous reconstructive surgery. Int Angiol 1985;4:455-62.
90. Sottiurai VS. Venous bypass and valve reconstruction: indication, technique and results. Phlebology 1997;25:183-8.
91. Kistner RL. Surgical repair of a venous valve. Straub Clin Proc 1968;34:41-3.
92. Perrin M. Reconstructive surgery for deep venous reflux: a report on 144 cases. Cardiovasc Surg 2000;8:246-55.
93. Masuda EM, Kirstner RL. Long term results of venous valve reconstruction: a 4 to 21 year follow up. J Vasc Surg 1994;19:391-403.
94. Kirstner RL. Surgical technique of external valve repair. Straub Found Proc 1990;55:15-6.
95. Gloviczki P, Merrel SW, Bower TC. Femoral vein valve repair under direct vision without venotomy: a modified technique with use of angioscopy. J Vasc Surg 1991;14:645-8.
96. Raju S, Bery MA, Neglen P. Transcommisural valvuloplasty: technique and results. J Vasc Surg 2000;32:969-76.
97. Hallberg D. A method for repairing incompetent valves in deep veins. Acta Chir Scand 1972;138:143-5.
98. Ferris EB, Kirstner RL. Femoral vein reconstruction in the management of chronic venous insufficiency. A 14 year experience. Arch Surg 1982;117:1571-9.
99. Raju S, Fredericks R. Valve reconstruction procedures for non obstructive venous insufficiency: rationale, techniques and results in 107 procedures with two to eight year follow up. J Vasc Surg 1988;7:301-10.

100. Bry JA, Muto PA, O'Donnell TF. The clinical and hemodynamic results after axillary to popliteal vein valve transplantation. J Vasc Surg 1995;21:110–9.
101. Wilson NM, Rutt DL, Browse ML. In situ venous valve construction. Br J Surg 1991;78:595–600.
102. Psathakis MD. The substitute "valve" operation by technique in patients with post thrombotic syndrome. Surgery 1984;95:542–8.
103. Raju S, Fredericks RK, Mezlem PM, et al. Durability of venous valve reconstruction techniques for primary and post thrombotic reflux. J Vasc Surg 1996;23: 357–67.

Endovascular Therapy for Limb Salvage

Michal Nawalany, MD

KEYWORDS

- Critical limb ischemia • Limb salvage • Percutaneous therapy
- Endovascular technology

Critical limb ischemia (CLI) is defined by the presence of rest pain, nonhealing ulceration, or gangrene plus objective evidence of diffuse pedal ischemia (Fontaine classes III and IV or Rutherford categories 4, 5, or 6).[1] CLI is an end stage of chronic insufficiency of blood supply to the lower extremity. Timely revascularization of ischemic limbs is crucial to limb salvage. Only 50% of CLI patients will remain amputation-free at 1 year, 25% will have a major amputation, and the remaining 25% will have died.[2] Without revascularization, patients with disease of Rutherford category 5 and 6 will have a 95% 1-year major amputation rate.[3]

CLI patients represent 1% of the 60 to 80 million Americans with peripheral arterial disease (PAD). These patients have an associated mortality of up to 70% at 5 years. Symptomatic patients with CLI have a 15-fold higher risk of dying of cardiovascular complications compared with the 3- to 6-fold higher risk for the asymptomatic population with PAD. This group of patients clearly is debilitated, and being a limb salvage surgeon requires an optimistic mindset. If successful, benefits to the patient are obvious. Societal benefits (of limb salvage) in terms of saved health care dollars are also well documented.[4]

Historically, limb salvage revascularization surgery meant laborious bypasses occasionally involving arm vein, spliced vein, composite grafts, or other heroic means to create a suitable conduit. Primary amputation was sometimes advised as a safer option. Percutaneous therapy has gradually been adopted as an alternative to primary amputation in persons deemed unsuitable as surgical candidates, and has established itself as a primary mode of treatment.[5,6] In recent years clinicians have witnessed an explosion in endovascular technology and a revolution in revascularization patterns for limb salvage. Open surgery is now frequently reserved for failure of endovascular attempts or pathology unsuitable for endovascular revascularization.[6] The purpose of this review is to educate the practicing general surgeon about the usefulness and appropriate application of different therapeutic endovascular options as applied to limb salvage.

Department of Vascular Surgery, Marshfield Clinic, 1000 North Oak Avenue, Marshfield, WI 54449, USA
E-mail address: Nawalany.michal@marshfieldclinic.org

Surg Clin N Am 90 (2010) 1215–1225
doi:10.1016/j.suc.2010.08.007
0039-6109/10/$ – see front matter © 2010 Elsevier Inc. All rights reserved.

Evaluation of a patient who presents with CLI includes proper history with inquiry about diabetes, renal function, heart disease, tobacco abuse, interval of nonhealing, prior ulcers, type of wound care received, vein harvest, and any previous revascularization. Persons at highest risks for severe vascular disease and limb loss are diabetics, those with renal failure, those of Afro-American heritage, or current smokers. Awareness of coexisting conditions helps with risk stratification and selection of the appropriate treatment option.

Vascular examination delineates the extent of ischemic tissue burden, rules out active limb-threatening infections, and assesses blood supply. Although no agreement exists as to what constitutes a nonsalvageable foot, primary amputation can and should be entertained in patients presenting with:

1. Extensive foot necrosis extending proximal to the metatarsal bones
2. Sepsis that involves the tarsal bones, ankle, or soft tissues of the calf with severe systemic illness
3. Debilitated and bedridden patients with no ambulatory potential.

Some of these patients will still require assessment of blood flow or revascularization to heal even more proximal amputations. Relatively few of the institutionalized or dependent patients regain their independence[7] but in functional patients presenting with CLI, the surgeon should be willing to invest time and effort to achieve improvement in blood flow and help tip the scale in favor of healing. However, the decision to proceed with limb salvage should not be made purely on the technical feasibility or dollar sense but should involve patient perceptions of quality of life, which do not always equate with prolonged wound healing.[7]

Evaluating blood flow and ensuring proper blood supply is one of the core principles when presented with a foot wound. Occasionally foot ulceration is seen in presence of palpable pedal pulses as a result of diseased microcirculation and neuropathy, but more commonly CLI is a result of multilevel disease and is a result of complex pathology related to chronic shortage of blood supply. Any patient presenting with CLI and absence of pedal pulses should undergo objective assessment of vascular supply. Noninvasive arterial studies consisting of an ankle-brachial index (ABI) with arterial waveforms should be obtained. Quality of the waveforms should be reviewed as the ABI will often be falsely elevated in this group of patients because of vessel calcification and incompressibility. Major procedures on a patient with a falsely elevated ABI may result in failure to achieve the desired healing and subject the patient to a higher than necessary level of amputation. Marston and colleagues[8] looked at the natural course of chronic leg ischemia in patients who could not undergo revascularization. An index of less than 0.5 was a significant predictor of amputation, with 28% and 34% of limbs experiencing limb loss at 6 and 12 months, respectively, compared with 10% and 15% of limbs in patients with an ABI of greater than 0.5 ($P<.01$). In 50% of limbs, however, ABI was not obtainable due to noncompressible vessels. A great proportion of the diabetic patients will fall into the latter category. The only predictor of healing was the initial wound size. Ballard and colleagues[9] documented successful healing with conservative care in 86% of limbs with transcutaneous oxygen ($TcPO_2$) levels greater than 30 mm Hg, including 73% (11 of 15) limbs without a palpable pulse. Usefulness of the transcutaneous oximetry in predicting healing potential has been contested, especially in the face of active infection or limb swelling, but the presence of low values (<20 mm Hg) should prompt more aggressive evaluation of circulation. For cases with a lesser disease burden in which blood supply seems to be robust even if not direct (lack of pulses) and $TcPO_2$ levels are higher than 40 mm Hg, it is reasonable to attempt a course of wound care or even minor amputations. Close follow-up is essential to detect deterioration and allow timely intervention. Major amputations should be deferred whenever possible until proper assessment of blood flow or revascularization has occurred. Of course, guillotine amputations for septic source containment are still performed without delay as deemed necessary by the patient's condition.

For feet with extensive ischemic burden or where significant amputations are likely, one should proceed with mapping of the blood supply without delay. Obtaining noninvasive studies is still useful in establishing baseline for the monitoring of effectiveness of therapy and follow-up.

Preoperative imaging in the form of computed tomographic angiography (CTA) or magnetic resonance angiography (MRA) allows for better case planning and has been found to be cost effective. Occasionally it spares the patient from an invasive procedure, alters the approach, or routes the patient toward a primary open surgical repair. Before imaging, renal function is checked. For those with borderline renal function, protective measures with hydration and bicarbonate infusion are instituted. In cases of critical renal impairment, imaging is still possible with time-of-flight MRA or CO_2 arteriography. Duplex can be fairly consistently used to map out the flow through the superficial femoral artery (SFA), but visualizing diseased tibial vessels is more challenging.

Direct angiography is still the gold standard and is often necessary before any attempts at vascular reconstruction. Diagnostic angiography is generally performed from the contralateral side via a retrograde common femoral approach. This approach allows evaluation of the inflow as well as the outflow in the affected limb. In cases of hostile groins or unfavorable aortic bifurcation (steep angle, prior bypass, or stents) it can also be done from a brachial approach.

Vessels are generally accessed where they can be easily compressed following catheter removal, such as the common femoral artery (CFA) over the femoral neck. For patients in whom disease is felt to reside in the distal SFA or the infrapopliteal location (eg, diabetics with present popliteal pulse), common femoral vessels can be accessed in an antegrade fashion. If there is any question about patency of the proximal SFA, duplex ultrasound can be used. Antegrade access allows more direct wire control as the tortuosity of the iliac system is removed. In tall patients it may be the only way to reach a very distal lesion. Antegrade access becomes challenging in obese individuals, as the size of the pannus readily interferes with introduction of the access catheter. Determining the exact point of compression after sheath removal is equally difficult, and may lead to postoperative hematomas. In general, access complications are fewer using a retrograde rather than an antegrade common femoral approach. Regular use of ultrasonography for access has been reported to reduce complication rates. The brachial approach limits the extent of therapeutic reach to the SFA (unless in persons of really short stature), mainly because of catheter length constraints. Brachial access has an associated risk of direct median nerve injury or palsy secondary to compression in the case of a hematoma. The brachial artery tends to roll away during compression and pseudoaneurysms are fairly common. There is also a risk of stroke, as the catheter will cross a vertebral artery coming from the left and the origins of both carotids coming from the right. For this reason the left brachial is more commonly used. It is important to check bilateral arm pressures before the procedure to avoid encountering an occult left subclavian artery occlusion. Any prior computed tomography studies of the chest should be reviewed to assess the degree of calcification within the aortic arch and to assess the degree of angulation at which the subclavian artery joins the aorta. Due to a higher risk of complication with brachial artery punctures, planned open exposure is sometimes done especially if a large sheath is to be used. In cardiology there is an increased interest in using the radial artery approach but, due to the size of the sheath and distance to lesion needed for peripheral interventions, it is less practical. One should not forget the option of direct exposure of the vessels elsewhere for endovascular therapy. Hostile groin can often be avoided by exposing the SFA in the proximal thigh, which can often be done with regional or local anesthesia in even the sickest patients. Infrapopliteal or even pedal vessels have been accessed in a retrograde fashion, with success for cases refractory to crossing in an antegrade fashion.

Vascular principles for endovascular surgery are the same as for open surgical procedures: ensure proper inflow before intervening on the outflow. Presence of strong femoral pulses is sufficient evidence of adequate inflow (it is usually supported by normal high thigh index or favorable waveforms). Diminished high thigh index may occasionally reflect disease in the proximal SFA rather than iliac vessels—so-called inflow equivalent. Although it is uncommon to have severe limb ischemia with isolated chronic inflow disease (unlike acute occlusion), the presence of significant inflow stenosis readily decreases global perfusion to the leg and should be corrected before further interventions down the leg. For superficial ulceration or rest pain, treatment of the inflow alone may prove sufficient to heal the wounds or resolve the pain.

Iliac vessels are readily available for percutaneous therapy. These vessels are generally large and easily reached. Access is fairly standard via the CFA. Lesions in the common iliac or proximal external iliac are frequently approached via ipsilateral CFA whereas those in the distal external iliac (close to the inguinal ligament) often use access from the contralateral side. Iliac vessels can also be reached via the brachial approach (although treatment is limited by the ability to deliver a large sheath from the arm and stent choices). While not universal,[10,11] use of stents is commonly accepted in the iliac circulation, as plaque tends to be extensive and have high recoil propensity. Providers dispute the advantages of balloon-expandable versus self-expanding stents in this vascular bed. Balloon-expandable stents generally are felt to have more radial strength, allowing primary stenting and more precise deployment, whereas the self-expandable stents are more adaptable to differences in diameter and may be more flexible. These stents generally require pre- or postdilatation of a lesion. Chang and colleagues[12] found hybrid treatment of iliac-femoral occlusive disease, consisting of common femoral endarterectomy and stenting/stent-grafting of the iliacs, to rival gold standard open aortofemoral repair and to outperform an extra-anatomic bypass. Perioperative mortality was 2.3%. Primary patency, assisted primary patency, and secondary patency were 60%, 97%, and 98% at 5 years. Stent grafts had statistically better patency than bare metal stents. Stenting alone in the presence of significant CFA disease had poorer outcomes and was recommended against. In another study, Timaran and colleagues[13] found external iliac occlusive disease, female gender, and presence of compromised runoff (occluded SFA) to be predictors of early stent failure, and recommended considering open surgical bypass in the above scenario. The use of covered stent grafts in the iliac vessels has its proponents, but clear superiority has not been demonstrated. Due to generally higher costs, they are often reserved for treating complications such as focal perforations or significant dissections. Occasionally they are also used to treat long occlusions (Trans Atlantic InterSociety Consensus [TASC] C or D) to minimize the intimal hyperplasia ingrowth into the stent.

The CFA is an area poorly suited for percutaneous intervention. Stenting is ill advised in this highly mobile area because of concerns about stent fracture. In addition, stenting the origin of the SFA risks compromising the flow through the profunda. The profunda artery should be protected, as it is often a source of limb-saving collateral blood flow in cases of SFA occlusion. Though usually not required, sending a buddy wire into the profunda and/or using kissing balloons when treating the origin of the SFA may sometimes be advisable. Vessel diameter and degree of plaque in the CFA usually exceeds the capabilities of current percutaneous atherectomy devices. Such attempts also carry a significant risk of distal embolization. The groin is usually easily accessible, under local anesthesia if needed, and therefore amenable to open plaque debulking even in high-risk patients. Significant disease here is usually treated with open endarterectomy with patch angioplasty. The open approach also allows simultaneous treatment of the very important profunda artery. Much like improvements of inflow, corrective surgery in the groin is often enough to reverse early ischemia without the need to reestablish direct blood flow to the foot. Open groin revascularization can be also coupled with endovascular treatment of the outflow. Improved endovascular salvage options also are responsible for renewed interest in remote endarterectomy (which fell out of favor because of high rates of early restenosis). Rosenthal and colleagues[14] reported primary assisted patency of 88.5% at 18 months for Aspire stent–assisted remote endarterectomy treatment of long occlusions of the SFA.

The majority of typical limb salvage surgery deals with improvement of the outflow circulation. Surgical bypass with vein remains the gold standard of repair against which all other modalities are compared. Data from the PREVENT III trial revealed a 2.7% perioperative mortality, 5.2% rate of graft occlusion, 16% mortality at 1 year, 80% secondary patency at 1 year, and 88% limb salvage rate at 1 year.[15]

Preoperative use of CTA/MRA has already been alluded to. Based on these studies, some patients may be routed toward an open bypass as a primary mode of revascularization, for example, TASC D occlusion, as recommended by the TASC II document. Another finding that leads some clinicians to an open first approach is that of a flush occlusion of the SFA. In these scenarios it is much more difficult to engage the plaque, as the wire has a tendency to slip into the patent profunda.

Percutaneous therapy largely depends on the ability to deliver the wire and subsequently a treatment catheter/balloon through the area of stenosis or occlusion. There is a multitude of wires ranging in gauge, stiffness, hydrophilicity, and shape, and an even greater choice of supporting catheters. Lyden[16] summarized the commonly employed techniques for crossing occlusions, but each interventionalist usually arrives at a functional combination of a wire and catheter that works well for him or her with respect to specific encountered pathology. For larger vessels, a 0.35-inch system usually suffices. For more stubborn occlusions, an angled guidewire is felt to be somewhat more able to maneuver through porosities. For infrapopliteal lesions a 0.014-inch or an 0.018-inch wire-based system maybe more useful. Details of techniques are beyond the scope of this article, but the interested reader is referred to the Schneider textbook titled *Endovascular Skills* as an excellent reference on all aspects of endovascular technique. For those with basic skills looking for more technical tips on dealing with tibial disease, the review by Blevins and Schneider[17] of endovascular CLI management is recommended.

Occlusions can be crossed intraluminally or subintimally (between the fused atherosclerosed intima-media layer and the adventitial wall). Patency rates are largely comparable using the 2 techniques in the SFA.[18] Subintimal crossing sometimes requires the usage of reentry catheters to redirect the wire intraluminally.[19] There are 2 reentry catheters available on the market. The Pioneer catheter (Medtronic Inc, Minneapolis, MN, USA) is a 7F intravascular ultrasound–oriented catheter, which uses a side-placed needle port to puncture back into the lumen. The Outback catheter (Cordis Corp, Miami Lakes, FL, USA) is a 5F angled catheter with a needle at the tip which, once the catheter is oriented toward the lumen, can be used to puncture through the dissection plane.

Crossing the lesion often constitutes the most difficult part of the procedure. Several technologies have been developed to aid crossing. The CROSSER device (Flow Cardia, Sunnyvale, CA, USA) is delivered to the area of occlusion over a standard guidewire. When the CROSSER catheter is activated using the foot switch, the Nitinol core wire transmits the vibrational energy to the metal tip of the catheter. The high-frequency mechanical vibration facilitates guidewire passage of the chronic total occlusion, much like a "micro jackhammer." This device is touted to aid crossing difficult lesions intraluminally and to cut down the time of crossing lesions overall.

When faced with an occlusion resistant to wire/catheter technique, another option is the use of the excimer laser. This laser employs photochemical, photothermal, and photomechanical mechanisms to ablate thrombus and plaque. The photochemical effect fractures tissue bonds within 100 μm of the catheter tip with each pulse of energy lasting 125 nanoseconds. The photothermal effect is caused by molecular vibration, with energy transfer leading to vaporization of plaque. The photomechanical effect is a result of the vapor bubble expanding and collapsing. The laser has been used with modified catheters to debulk plaque, but its greatest value probably lies in the ability to cross an occlusion without a leading wire.

Treatment is usually performed with appropriate level of anticoagulation (activated clotting time >250 seconds) as well as antecedent usage of dual antiplatelet therapy in the form of Plavix (clopidrogel bisulfate) and aspirin to help minimize risk of immediate thrombosis either at or distal to the site of angioplasty. Balloon angioplasty remains the most common method of treatment and the percutaneous standard against which all new technology is tested. This technique has withstood the test of time well, and in comparison with newer more tech-savvy devices is extremely cost effective. With respect to original devices, balloons have become progressively sleeker and packaged into lower profile catheters, allowing easier crossing and treatment of even small tibial vessels; they are also available in a greater variety of lengths. Over-the-wire balloons can be used as a support catheter, whereas monorail balloons speed up catheter exchange and can be used for treatment provided the delivery path is free of obstacles. The balloon is usually initially slightly undersized with respect to the diameter of the vessel. Multiple insufflations using progressively larger balloons are sometimes necessary to achieve the desired effect. The general recommendation is for the final angioplasty to be done with a balloon 1 mm larger than the diameter of the vessel to accommodate for healing reactions that will take place following angioplasty. In tibial vessels, Blevins and Schneider[17] recommend using an appropriate-size balloon without oversizing. In general, aggressive oversizing creates a higher risk of dissections or vessel rupture. The former can be treated by reangioplasty with prolonged balloon inflation or coverage with a stent. Covered stents (stent grafts) can be used to rescue a ruptured vessel. In general, covered stents require larger delivery sheaths than their bare metal equivalents, and are more expensive. Cutting balloons are specialized balloons with blades inserted into the balloon. These devices carry a higher risk of vessel perforation, are inflated slowly, and generally are under-sized by 1 mm with respect to the actual lumen of the vessel. Although some groups use them for treatment of primary lesions and claim improved results,[20] the majority believes they are most suitable for reangioplasty, where stenosis is more likely caused by intimal hyperplasia. Cutting balloons are also used by some clinicians for the treatment of vein graft stenosis.

Once a lesion has been crossed with a wire, a multitude of other therapeutic options exist. The SFA is the focus of the greatest variety of options. Vessels are of medial diameter and rupture rarely results in life-threatening emergency, therefore aggressive approaches are often tried. Revascularization options here include anything from conventional balloon angioplasty (either transluminal or subintimal), bare metal versus covered stents, atherectomy/debulking, and cryoplasty to a totally percutaneous extravascular bypass.[21]

Although there are data to suggest superiority of stenting in the SFA over balloon angioplasty alone in terms of vessel patency and relief of symptoms at 6 and 12 months,[22] it is by no means universally accepted and does not confer long-term patency advantage. In general, very little to no randomized or high-class data exist to establish clear superiority of one form of treatment over another. Studies mix patients treated for claudication with those treated for limb salvage, lesions treated in the SFA with those in the infrageniculate circulation or mixed, and many are tainted by industry support or involvement.

In the absence of widely accepted randomized data, some simple ideas help define the optimal treatment. In general, for longer occlusions (TASC C and D) stents may be advantageous in prolonging the primary patency interval. This short-term patency advantage may be very important in getting a lesion to heal before restenosis. For lesions in the TASC A or B, such an advantage is less clear. Lesions with a good response to percutaneous transluminal angioplasty (PTA) (<20% restenosis) may be observed.

Some clinicians are in favor of covered stent grafts for lining very long occlusions, in essence creating an internal polytetrafluoroethylene bypass. Kedora and colleagues[23] compared in a randomized fashion the use of stent grafts with a prosthetic bypass, and found comparable primary patency of both at slightly over 70% at 1 year. Covered stent grafts fail at the ends but are free from intimal ingrowth throughout the graft, and may be easier to rescue. Atherectomy may be a good option for a small, very heavily calcified SFA resistant to high-pressure balloon angioplasty. No meaningful benefit in terms of improved patency has been shown by atherectomy versus less expansive balloon angioplasty.[24] Atherectomy may also be useful in the treatment of lesions in the popliteal artery where dissections are less easily correctable by stenting, or in the treatment of small tibial vessels.

Popliteal artery, much like the CFA, spans a highly mobile area of the knee joint. Stenting here with conventional bare metal stents may lead to fracture, with prolonged flexion and higher risk of thrombosis. Ultraflexible stents and grafts offer some encouraging results. Recent meta-analysis of stent grafting for popliteal artery aneurysm showed the stent grafts to carry comparable patency to open repair, with primary patency of 83% at 1 year (95% confidence interval [CI], 79%–88%) and at 3 years primary patency of 74% (95% CI, 67%–81%) and secondary patency of 85% (95% CI, 78%–91%).[17] In another report fractures were identified in 16.7% of stents, with the majority occurring at the site of stent overlap, but no difference in patency was observed.[25] Caution has to be exercised in extrapolating these data from very carefully selected patients with good runoff to critical ischemia and limb salvage.

Tibial vessels represent the biggest challenge for limb salvage surgeons. Open surgery below the knee requires the presence of vein for meaningful patency of a bypass, and this often becomes a limiting factor in this group of patients who might have had vein harvested, either for cardiac or previous peripheral interventions. The other factor, of course, is the overall fitness of the patient to withstand a prolonged operation. Tibial vessels are small, usually heavily calcified, and do not lend themselves well to subintimal interventions. Long segment occlusions are the norm.

Operating here requires a working expertise as well as knowledge of the properties of different wires and catheters. These vessels are prone to distal embolization and acute thrombosis. It is in this area where the emerging technology may make the biggest impact. Percutaneous therapy allows minimally invasive treatment of crucial vessels. Poor patency, measured in months (<40% at 1 year), is offset by reproducibility of the procedures.

Complications of endovascular therapy are grouped into access, direct vessel injury, and others. Pseudoaneurysm should be suspected with pain in the groin in excess of what is expected. Patients often describe "a pop in the groin." Pulsatile mass in the groin suggests a pseudoaneurysm, and duplex is a confirmatory study of choice. Small pseudoaneurysms may resolve with observation. People on chronic anticoagulation require closer consideration of definitive open repair. Those with a long narrow neck may be treated percutaneously with thrombin injection. Presence of an arteriovenous fistula or suspicion of infection is a contraindication to injecting thrombin. Infections are relatively uncommon and usually occur in a setting of significant hematomas or closure devices; they may need to be treated with open debridement and reconstruction of the vessel wall.

In addition to perforations and dissections that are relatively easily dealt with in most locations, distal embolization can be problematic. Several aspiration catheters exist and are the authors' first choice for treatment. Occasionally reangioplasty or thrombolysis (if a platelet clump is suspected) can be helpful. One must always ensure that the level of anticoagulation is adequate before treatment. The second rule of thumb is to maintain wire access through the area being treated until absolutely sure the procedure is finished. The tip of the wire should always be visible at the bottom of the screen. If the tip travels too deep it can lead to perforation, vascular spasm, or coil, and lead to thrombosis of outflow vessels.

Anaphylactoid reactions are uncommon with proper questioning about contrast hypersensitivity. Contrast nephrotoxicity is more frequently encountered in this group of patients. For patients with elevated creatinine or history of renal insufficiency the authors use periprocedural hydration and bicarbonate infusion. Risks of nephrotoxicity are disclosed preoperatively, and renal function closely followed postoperatively.

Much concern has been raised about endovascular therapy hindering subsequent successful bypass revascularization. Joels and colleagues[26] found that early failures of percutaneous SFA therapy were usually amenable to percutaneous recanalization, with a secondary patency rate of 76%. The surgical bypass site was altered in 6 limbs (28.6%); 4 from popliteal to tibial and 2 from above-knee to below-knee popliteal. Only 1 of 276 limbs required an amputation (0.04%). On the other hand, endovascular therapy sometimes allows limb salvage following a failed bypass. Looking at patients with a failed bypass and ischemic lower extremity and excluding patients with percutaneous attempts at reopening the bypass, Simosa and colleagues[27] identified 24 limbs in 23 patients whose limbs were salvaged by percutaneous therapy for the native circulation. Multifocal lesions were identified (87% had TASC C and D lesions) but investigators had 100% technical success rate. Some limbs needed reangioplasty and some went on to a secondary bypass. Four amputations were noted. Results for PTA were 72% secondary patency rate and 81% rate of limb salvage at 3 years.

In general, caution is recommended in stenting areas that eliminate a potential bypass landing zone and commit a patient to a more distal bypass. If a patient really is not an open surgical candidate, this may be less of a concern. By far the biggest complication and reason for failure of initially successful endovascular therapy is lack of appropriate follow-up, at least until the wounds are completely healed. The authors' protocol consists of either immediate postoperative ABI/duplex or initial study within 2 weeks of intervention followed by 1-, 3-, 6-, 9-, and 12-month studies, then 6 months × 2, and yearly. According to a recent meta-analysis, the primary average patency of percutaneous interventions is 77% at 1 month, 58% at 1 year, and 48% at 3 years versus bypass 93%, 81%, and 72%, respectively. The limb salvage rates, however, did not differ as significantly: 93%, 86%, 82% versus 95%, 88%, 82%.

At the 2009 Society for Vascular Surgery conference, attendees were anonymously polled with respect to appropriate management of a TASC D lesion, and most chose open surgery. Despite this, the majority said that in practice they would attempt an endovascular approach first. Reasons may include lesser morbidity, absence of contraindications, and open approach still available as a rescue in most situations. This answer may also be partially reflective of reimbursement patterns, as 1 hour of endovascular work pays more than an hour of open surgical time.

Lawrence and Chandra[28] polled 5 prominent "endo first" (but dual trained) surgeons as to what parameters would make them consider open surgery as initial therapy. Five factors were based on anatomy, pathology, physiology, durability, and limited distal targets:

1. Disease of the CFA—due to extent of plaque and size of vessels exceeding current atherectomy devices as well as ease of open surgical accessibility and durability of repair
2. Extrinsic compression—endovascular repair does not eliminate pathology related to, for example, popliteal entrapment or cystic disease
3. Extensive foot sepsis/widespread tissue involvement—despite absence of level I data, the general feeling is that open surgical procedures result in more pulsatile flow and therefore should be considered in these situations to minimize tissue loss
4. Young patients or those treated with a transfer flap were felt to need the most durable approach
5. Single distal target vessel was felt to be a relative contraindication to endovascular approach for the fear of embolization and target loss.

In their treatment algorithm, Blevins and Schneider[17] felt that endovascular therapy is most useful when applied early, when tissue loss is impending or developing rather than when extensive ischemic insult with gangrene has occurred. For extensive disease in a fit patient with suitable target and conduit, open surgical bypass was still recommended as the treatment of choice. If the endovascular route was chosen (especially in the face of significant ischemic burden), an attempt at opening all vessels was suggested.

In conclusion, endovascular surgery can be applied with comparable rates of limb salvage to a wide spectrum of patients with CLI and can spare them from the increased morbidity of open repairs. Furthermore, endovascular surgery offers a minimally invasive option to revascularize individuals previously felt suitable only for primary amputations. Properly applied endovascular surgery does not preclude subsequent open repair and can be complementary: via bypass salvage, improving inflow or outflow, or limb salvage following a failed bypass. Hybrid use of open and endovascular approaches may benefit the patient by providing the necessary improvements in blood flow and limiting morbidity. The patient's best interest should always be the top priority in decision making. There is a need for randomized control trials to define specific patient characteristics to find out exactly who benefits most from an endo versus open approach, in terms of individual patient gains and patient-perceived improvements in quality of life, as well as societal cost reduction. There is a similar need to compare various percutaneous modalities and to evaluate the durability of percutaneous interventions that use expensive new technology. Limb salvage rates generally exceed the patency rates of percutaneous interventions, but close postoperative surveillance is critical to successful limb salvage, at least until full healing is achieved.

REFERENCES

1. Varu VN, Hogg ME, Kibbe MR. Critical limb ischemia. J Vasc Surg 2010;51: 230–41.
2. Norgren L, Hiatt WR, Dormandy JA, et al. Inter-society consensus for the management of peripheral arterial disease (TASC II). Eur J Vasc Endovasc Surg 2007;20:62–7.
3. Wolfe JH, Wyatt MG. Critical and subcritical ischaemia. Eur J Vasc Endovasc Surg 1997;13:578–82.
4. Singh S, Evens L, Datta D, et al. The costs of managing lower limb-threatening ischaemia. Eur J Vasc Endovasc Surg 1996;12:359–62.
5. Tefera G, Hoch J, Turnipseed W. Limb salvage angioplasty in vascular surgery practice. J Vasc Surg 2005;41:988–93.
6. Kudo T, Chandra F, Kwun WH, et al. Changing pattern of surgical revascularization for critical limb ischemia over 12 years: endovascular vs open bypass surgery. J Vasc Surg 2006;44:304–13.
7. Nehler MR, Haitt WR, Taylor LM. Is revascularization and limb salvage always the best treatment for critical limb ischemia? J Vasc Surg 2003;37:704–8.
8. Marston WA, Davies SW, Armstrong B, et al. Natural history of limbs with arterial insufficiency and chronic ulceration treated without revascularization. J Vasc Surg 2006;44:108–14.
9. Ballard JL, Eke CJ, Bunt TJ, et al. A prospective evaluation of transcutaneous oxygen measurements in the evaluation of diabetic foot problems. J Vasc Surg 1995;22:485–92.
10. Kudo T, Chandra FA, Ahn SS. Long term outcomes and predictors of iliac angioplasty with selective stenting. J Vasc Surg 2005;42:466–75.
11. Kang JL, Patel VI, Conrad MF, et al. Common femoral artery occlusive disease: contemporary results following surgical endarterectomy. J Vasc Surg 2008;48: 872–7.
12. Chang R, Goodney P, Baek J, et al. Long term results of combined common femoral endarterectomy and iliac stenting/stent grafting for occlusive disease. J Vasc Surg 2008;48:362–7.
13. Timaran C, Prault T, Stevens S, et al. Iliac artery stenting versus surgical reconstruction for TASC type B and type C iliac lesions. J Vasc Surg 2003;38:272–8.
14. Rosenthal D, Martin JD, Schubart PI, et al. Remote superficial femoral artery endarterectomy and distal aspire stents multicenter medium term results. J Vasc Surg 2004;40:67–72.
15. Conte MS, Bandyk DF, Clowes AW, et al. Results of prevent III: multicenter randomized trial of edifoligide for the prevention of vein graft failure in lower extremity bypass surgery. J Vasc Surg 2006;43:742–50.
16. Lyden SP. Techniques and outcomes for endovascular treatment in the tibial arteries. J Vasc Surg 2009;50:1219–23.
17. Blevins WA, Schneider PA. Endovascular management of critical limb ischemia. Eur J Vasc Endovasc Surg 2010;39:756–61.

18. Antusevas A, Aleksynos N, Kaupas RS, et al. Comparison of results of subintimal angioplasty and percutaneous transluminal angioplasty in SFA occlusions. Eur J Vasc Endovasc Surg 2008;36:101–6.
19. Jacobs DL, Motaganahalli RL, Cox DE, et al. True lumen reentry devices facilitate subintimal angioplasty and stenting of total chronic occlusions. J Vasc Surg 2006; 43:1291–6.
20. Canaud L, Aric P, Berthet JP, et al. Infrainguinal cutting balloons in de novo arterial lesions. J Vasc Surg 2008;48:1182–6.
21. Wagner JK, Chaer RA, Rhea RY, et al. True lumen re entry after extra vascular recanalization of SFA for chronic total occlusion. J Vasc Surg 2010;32:216–8.
22. Schillinger M, Sabeti S, Loewe C, et al. Balloon angioplasty vs implantation of nitinol stents in the SFA. N Engl J Med 2006;354:1879–88.
23. Kedora J, Hohmann S, Garrett W, et al. Randomized comparison of percutaneous Viabahn stent graft vs prosthetic femoral popliteal bypass in the treatment of superficial femoral artery occlusive disease. J Vasc Surg 2007;45(1):10–6.
24. White CJ, Gray WA. Endovascular therapy for peripheral arterial disease: an evidence based review. Circulation 2007;116:2203–15.
25. Trelliu IF, Zeebregts CJ, Varliotakis G, et al. Stent fractures in the Hemobahn/Viabahn stent graft after endovascular popliteal aneurysm repair. J Vasc Surg 2010; 51:1413–8.
26. Joels CS, York JW, Kalbaugh CA, et al. Surgical implications of early failed endovascular intervention of the superficial femoral artery. J Vasc Surg 2008;47:562–5.
27. Simosa HF, Malek JY, Schermerhorn ML, et al. Endoluminal intervention for limb salvage after failed lower extremity bypass graft. J Vasc Surg 2009;49:1426–30.
28. Lawrence PF, Chandra A. When should open surgery be the initial option for critical limb ischaemia? Eur J Vasc Endovasc Surg 2010;39:S32–37.

Intra-abdominal Healing: Gastrointestinal Tract and Adhesions

Sanjay Munireddy, MD, Sandra L. Kavalukas, PA-C,
Adrian Barbul, MD*

KEYWORDS

• Anastomotic wound healing • Adhesion formation

The abdominal cavity represents one of the most active areas of surgical activity. Surgical procedures involving the gastrointestinal (GI) tract are among the most common procedures performed nowadays. Healing of the GI tract after removal of a segment of bowel and healing of the peritoneal surfaces with subsequent adhesion formation remain vexing clinical problems. Both represent aspects of wound healing and opportunities for either wound failure, such as in anastomotic leaks, or an over-zealous response as represented by clinically significant adhesions. Interventions to modify both the responses are myriad, yet a full understanding of the pathophysiology of these responses remains elusive. Such progress is of great interest because complications of abdominal healing represent a significant clinical and economic burden.[1–4]

HEALING IN THE GI TRACT
Anatomy

The GI tract wall, except for the esophagus and distal rectum, consists of 4 layers: mucosa, submucosa, muscularis propria, and serosa.[5] Mucosa, the innermost layer, is made of 3 sublayers: epithelium (generally columnar cells), lamina propria (containing blood vessels, lymphatics, mesenchymal cells, and inflammatory cells), and muscularis mucosa (thin smooth muscle layer). Injury caused to mucosa during anastomoses is repaired by migration and proliferation of epithelial cells, thus sealing the defect and creating a barrier to luminal contents.[6] Direct mucosal apposition is important for this process to occur quickly (as short as 3 days) as compared with mucosal eversion or inversion.[7] Submucosa is the most important layer of the

Department of Surgery, Sinai Hospital of Baltimore, and the Johns Hopkins Medical Institutions, Baltimore, MD, USA
* Corresponding author. Department of Surgery, Sinai Hospital of Baltimore, 2435 West Belvedere Avenue, Baltimore, MD 21215.
E-mail address: abarbul@jhmi.edu

Surg Clin N Am 90 (2010) 1227–1236
doi:10.1016/j.suc.2010.08.002
0039-6109/10/$ – see front matter

intestinal wall for surgeons because it provides most of the tensile strength and is the anchor for holding anastomotic sutures.[8] The submucosa consists of loose connective tissue containing the bulk of the structural collagen, nerve fibers, ganglia, blood, and lymphatic vessels. Predominant collagen is type I (68%), followed by types II (20%) and V (12%).[9] The muscularis propria consists of inner circular and outer longitudinal layers of smooth muscle cells intermingled with collagen fibers. The serosa is the outermost layer in the GI tract and is made of connective tissue containing mesothelial cells, blood vessels, and lymphatics. Parts of the GI tract that lack serosa (esophagus and distal rectum) are at an increased risk of leakage.

Physiology of Wound Healing

If the mucosa is the only injured layer, it heals by rapid epithelial cell proliferation and differentiation, in a process called epithelial restitution. Mesothelial (serosal) and mucosal healing can occur without scarring. However, full-thickness injuries require additional repair mechanisms involving nonepithelial cell populations and inflammatory processes[10] that provoke fibroblastic responses leading to scar formation.

Similar to cutaneous healing, the first phase of GI healing begins with hemostasis. Initial vasoconstriction is followed by vasodilation and increased vessel permeability (induced by kinins), which allows inflammatory cells (polymorphonuclear leukocytes) to diapedese into the wound. Diapedesis marks the beginning of the inflammatory phase, which is also characterized by edema formation, mainly in the subepithelial region of the mucosa and the submucosa[11]; edema can persist for up to 2 weeks. Neutrophils are the predominant cells during the first 24 hours and macrophages predominate after 48 hours, synthesizing and releasing growth factors that begin and amplify the healing response.[5,12] As mentioned, formation of a fibrin seal on the serosal side and serosal healing are essential for quickly achieving a watertight seal; the significantly higher rates of anastomotic failure observed clinically in segments of bowel that are extraperitoneal and lack serosa (ie, the esophagus and rectum) underscore the importance of this response. The early integrity of the anastomosis also depends on the suture-holding capacity of the intestinal wall, particularly of the submucosal layer.

The beginning of the proliferative phase is marked by the appearance of granulation tissue in the anastomotic wound. During the proliferative phase, collagen undergoes both synthesis (by smooth muscle cells and fibroblasts in the submucosal layer[13]) and lysis (by collagenase activity). Smooth muscle cells contribute more to absolute collagen formation than fibroblasts.[12] Collagen lysis caused by collagenase activity contributes to low anastomotic strength seen early after the formation of an anastomosis.[13,14] Thus, the anastomosis is at risk for leakage or dehiscence during the first 3 to 10 days. Gradually, fibroblasts and smooth muscle cells begin to synthesize collagen, which gradually strengthens the anastomosis. Clearly, any factor that enhances collagen lysis or decreases its synthesis results in a longer-lasting weak anastomosis, which is at greater risk for failure (**Fig. 1**).

The epithelial layer is fully reconstituted, after 1 to 2 weeks, over a submucosal granulomatous network consisting of proliferating smooth muscle cells and fibroblasts.[15] The final phase of healing involves maturation and remodeling of the collagenous network, which results in the anastomosis becoming thinner but stronger.

Measuring GI Healing

Most information on the mechanical characteristics of anastomoses is derived from animal studies; the relevance of the information, particularly in regard to the time line of the response, may vary widely from clinical practice, but its importance

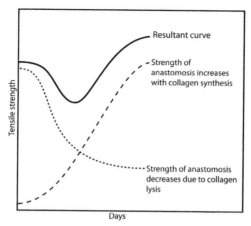

Fig. 1. The contribution of anastomotic collagen synthesis and lysis to overall anastomotic strength.

regarding validation of biologic principles should not be underestimated. Quantitative methods (mechanical and biochemical) have been described to assess the anastomotic strength of GI healing. Mechanical methods include breaking strength (measures longitudinal forces) and bursting pressure (measures intraluminal forces).[16] Breaking strength is a measure of the resistance of the intestinal wall against forces applied in longitudinal direction to the anastomosis.[15] Breaking strength is regained at a slower pace than bursting pressure and is 50% that of a normal colon at 10 days after injury.[17,18] Breaking strength is not sensitive enough to measure early changes in anastomotic healing.[15] Use of breaking strength has been criticized, because it is difficult to apply an equally distractive force in a circular direction to the circumference of the intestinal wall.[19] Bursting pressure is the intraluminal pressure at which the anastomosis disrupts. In animals, the intraluminal pressure is lowest during the first 3 days after anastomosis formation and, thereafter, it increases progressively. It is 50% of normal at 2 to 3 days and approaches 100% at 7 days.[5] Bursting pressure is, thus, a useful approach to measure changes in healing during the first week after creation of an anastomosis. Biochemical methods include measuring collagen deposition either by determining hydroxyproline content (an amino acid found almost exclusively in collagen) or by direct measurements; histologic and immunohistochemical methods have also been used.

Factors Affecting GI Wound Healing

Many factors have been implicated as having an effect on anastomotic healing and they can be classified as either systemic or local (**Table 1**). Some of the most common factors are discussed in the following sections.

Tissue perfusion

Intestinal mucosa is exquisitely sensitive to ischemia, which in the GI tract, rapidly becomes transmural and irreversible.[20] Restoration of blood flow to the ischemic bowel segment leads to reperfusion injury causing further tissue damage that frequently exceeds the boundaries of the original ischemic insult.[21] Thus, anastomoses created soon after the onset of reperfusion have a high failure rate. Adequate oxygen is a prerequisite for the hydroxylation of lysine and proline residues and critical

Table 1
Factors associated with negative effects on GI anastomotic healing

Factors	Local	Systemic
Intrinsic	Anastomotic tension Tissue hypoperfusion Local infection	Hypovolemia/shock Sepsis Immunodeficiency
Extrinsic	Radiation injury Bowel preparation	Blood transfusion Medications Malnutrition

for optimal collagen cross-linking and optimal collagen synthesis.[22] Mature collagen formation fails when tissue Po_2 is less than 40 mm Hg, and angiogenesis, epithelialization, and growth factors are impaired when tissue Po_2 is less than 10 mm Hg.[5] Ischemia-reperfusion injury is a systemic phenomenon, and even with remote organ so affected, anastomotic healing can be impaired.[22] In animal models, therapeutic modalities used successfully to decrease the deleterious effects of ischemia-reperfusion injury include ischemic preconditioning; therapy with hyperbaric oxygen, antioxidants, anticomplements, antileukocytes, perfluorocarbons; and nitric oxide (NO) and glutamine/glycine supplementation.[21]

Anemia had been implicated in the past as a factor contributing to anastomotic failure. However, anemia per se does not impair healing as long as sufficient tissue perfusion is maintained through maintenance of euvolemia and cardiac output.[12] Patients with good cardiac output can tolerate hematocrit levels down to 15%, as demonstrated by patients who refuse transfusion for religious principles.[23]

Acute hemorrhage can affect anastomotic bursting strength because of hypoproteinemia, factor XIII or vitamin C deficiency, and disturbances in coagulation.[24]

Nutrition

Wound healing requires adequate provision of energy and substrate. Numerous experimental and clinical studies demonstrate the detrimental effects of either short- or long-term malnutrition on anastomotic healing, although the exact mechanisms of action are not fully understood. Experimental studies demonstrate greater incidence of anastomotic dehiscence in malnourished rats and stronger intestinal anastomoses with increased intestinal suture-holding capacity in well-nourished rats.[25] Malnourished patients may lack cofactors required for collagen synthesis, such as vitamins A, C, and B6; zinc; and copper.[26] Malnutrition, also, causes deterioration in patients' immunocompetence with a higher risk of intra-abdominal or wound infection.

Intraperitoneal infection

Presence of infection in the abdominal cavity impairs anastomotic healing. Intra-abdominal sepsis results in decreased collagen formation at the anastomosis and significant decreases in bursting pressure.[27] Decreased collagen content at the anastomosis during peritonitis can be caused by decreased synthesis or increased breakdown of collagen. Increased breakdown is caused by bacterial collagenases from the peritoneal cavity or neutrophil collagenases from the increased inflammatory reaction during peritonitis.[12] Peritonitis, also, alters collagen gene expression, causing decreased collagen synthesis. Thus, intestinal anastomoses are at increased risk for leak or dehiscence in the presence of intra-abdominal sepsis, and most surgeons avoid construction of anastomoses in the face of peritonitis.

Radiation

Radiation is being used increasingly, in the perioperative period, to treat GI malignancies and its use has led to concerns regarding healing capacity of anastomosis. In animals, there is an early decrease in blood flow to the anastomotic area of the intestine, leading to complications.[28] However, localized preoperative irradiation does not compromise anastomotic healing in early postoperative period.[29] It is hypothesized that if radiation is given before the arrival of macrophages into the anastomotic wound, a normal healing cascade occurs.[29]

Blood transfusion

Blood transfusions adversely affect intestinal anastomotic healing in experimental animals.[30] Current thinking associates the immunosuppressive effects of blood transfusion with impaired healing. Leukocytes have been implicated to be responsible for immunosuppression-related defective healing and infectious complications because leukocyte-depleted blood transfusions have been shown to not cause such complications.[30] Transfusions, also, inhibit interleukin (IL) 2 production, thereby slowing the healing process.[31]

Mechanical bowel preparation

The practice of bowel cleansing before colorectal surgery has become a surgical dogma, and primary colonic anastomosis is traditionally considered unsafe in the face of an unprepared bowel. Although associated initially with reduced rates of surgical wound infections, the effect of bowel preparation regimens on anastomotic healing remains in doubt. Some animal studies have shown that mechanical preparation improved anastomotic bursting strength and decreased septic complications,[32] whereas other studies have failed to find a difference.[33–35]

Peritoneal Healing

Intra-abdominal adhesions are bands of scar tissue that form between loops of bowel and the abdominal wall. Adhesions have been identified as the cause of chronic pain and constipation since the late nineteenth century. During that period, scientists and physicians were aware that adhesions were caused by previous surgery, and the presumed cause was bacteriologic.[36] Medicine has come a long way in studying the molecular environment of the peritoneum and the many pathways that come into play during adhesion formation, and today the bacteriologic theory has been discarded. However, many theories including ischemia, immunologic abnormalities, surgical trauma and technical handling of tissues, hemorrhage, foreign bodies, and pathways of inflammation remain current. The fibrinolytic pathway that occurs in the abdominal cavity after surgery has been under investigation since 1965 and continues to be extensively studied.[37,38]

The effect of this healing anomaly is significant and can lead to severe morbidity and mortality. It has been estimated that in 1994, approximately $1.3 billion were spent on hospital costs for abdominal surgeries related to adhesions.[39] It should be noted that this figure did not include the conservative management and medical admissions for small bowel obstruction for which intravenous hydration, nasogastric suction, and possibly parenteral nutrition were given without surgical intervention. Because most small bowel obstructions caused by adhesions resolve with medical therapy, one can only imagine the costs that were not extrapolated during this study. A more recent review approximates that in 2006, 2.7 million people underwent laparotomy for digestive or gynecologic indications.[40] Midgut and hindgut surgery result in a higher incidence of adhesion formation, whereas open laparotomy consistently has a higher incidence of adhesions compared with the laparoscopic equivalent in all surgeries except appendectomy.[40]

The morbidity related to adhesions is caused by tethering of viscera to either nearby organs or the abdominal wall causing the kinking of essentially a hollow tube. Adhesions are fibrous scars that form on the outside of the intestinal serosa, and when they are dense and unforgiving, the intestine may become obstructed (partially or completely). The twisting of the intestinal segment may result from being bound to the abdominal wall or other loops of bowel. Once any degree of obstruction occurs, the intestinal segment becomes distended, resulting in colicky pain. If the obstruction continues, nausea, vomiting, and obstipation may result. Worse still, if the obstruction involves a closed loop with closure of venous outflow, ischemia may result in loss of bowel viability and sepsis if not relieved early. This phenomenon can involve female reproductive organs, with adhesions causing deformity and blockage of the fallopian tube and fimbriae opening, resulting in either hydrosalpinx leading to chronic pelvic pain or infertility by inhibiting the capture of the egg released into the abdominal cavity.

The peritoneal environment is instrumental in the response to injury that occurs with surgery. The peritoneum is composed of mesothelial cells that respond to surgically induced tissue trauma, ischemia, and infection. The initial response involves migration and activation of macrophages in the peritoneum. Fibroblasts, platelets, and chemoattractants such as thrombin and plasmin are part of the cascade for healing and functional restoration. Vascular injury and subsequent endothelial cell activation result in fibrinogen accumulation and chemokine release.[41] Resident peritoneal macrophages migrate to the GI lymphoid tissue and express the P-selectin receptor that binds to the P-selectin glycoprotein ligand 1, which further attracts and activates other macrophages to the site of injury.[42]

Mast cells recruited secondary to the peritoneal trauma release histamine and vasoactive kinins, which in turn increases capillary permeability.[43] The resulting fibrinous exudate coats the outer serosa of the abdominal viscera and causes organs to adhere to each other. This process can occur in as little as 3 to 4 hours after the initial injury.[44,45] The proteinaceous exudate provides the scaffold for cellular migration, fibrin matrix formation, and activation of the fibrinolytic pathway.

Fibrinolysis occurs through the interaction of tissue plasminogen activator and uroplasminogen activator (uPA). These enzymes are responsible for degradation of fibrin, which can lead to the resolution of the early and flimsy fibrin-based adhesions. During normal homeostasis, plasminogen activator inhibitors (PAIs) 1 and 2 act to counterbalance the degradation of fibrin (**Fig. 2**). In abnormal healing, the inhibitors may predominate leading to further organization of the fibrin matrix with angiogenesis, influx of fibroblasts, and collagen synthesis, all resulting in fibrous adhesions.[46]

Because of the significant morbidity associated with adhesion formation, great efforts have been made to devise a means of preventing adhesions. Intra-abdominal ischemic and infectious processes are present in only a small percentage of cases and as such are unavoidable. However, injury from laparotomy remains the sole inciting factor most of the time, even with a single surgical intervention. Therefore, most investigations involve some treatment at the time of the initial surgery as a means of preventing adhesions.

The present emphasis of adhesion research is on the biomolecular pathways that are understood to be involved in adhesion formation. A more thorough and detailed understanding of these pathways forms the basis for devising preventive therapies. Transforming growth factor (TGF) β has been studied most extensively owing to its role as a profibrotic cytokine. TGF-β1 and 3 are found intraperitoneally on organ surfaces, with the isoform 1 being most often associated to tissue fibrosis. In addition,

Peritoneal injury

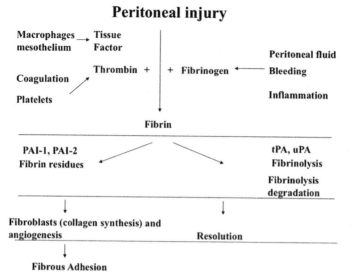

Fig. 2. Biochemical and cellular cascade occurring after peritoneal injury and leading to either consolidation or resorption of adhesions. tPA, tissue plasminogen activator.

TGF-β downregulates uPA and upregulates PAI-1, thus further increasing fibrotic organization.[41]

The role of macrophages in abdominal wound healing and adhesion formation has also been the focus of intensive research. Peritoneal macrophages are the predominant peritoneal cell type during adhesion formation.[47] Mice depleted of macrophages before abdominal wound formation showed significantly higher adhesion formation than nondepleted controls.[48] This result may be postulated to be because of a deficiency in uPA, tPA, and other vital chemokines secreted by macrophages. Macrophages downregulate fibroblast proliferation in the first 48 hours (key time of adhesion development) through prostaglandin E_2 and other fibroblast growth inhibitors, whereas later they stimulate fibroblast proliferation via the production and release of TGF-β and IL-1.[43]

More recently, the possible role of NO interacting with myeloperoxidase has been postulated and examined. An ischemic environment during peritoneal injury results in free radicals and NO production. Myeloperoxidase and NO seem to have a concerted role in both collagen deposition and possible downregulation of apoptosis in adhesions.[49]

Clinical approaches to the prevention of adhesions involve the use of physical barriers to decrease tissue apposition during the immediate postoperative period. By placing a film, gel, or other substance in the peritoneal cavity, which coats the bowel wall, an interference with fibrin matrix formation is achieved. A recent overview summarizes the different modalities available, ranging from carboxymethylcellulose, sodium hyaluronate, polyethylene glycol, and icodextrin.[50] The most used clinical products are Seprafilm (sodium hyaluronate; Genzyme Corp, Cambridge, MA, USA) and SurgiWrap (polylactic acid; MAST Biosurgery Inc, San Diego, CA, USA), both are available as sheets and applied directly to the undersurface of the incision. The main drawback with these and other products is their detrimental effect on bowel anastomoses. A study using a hyaluronate-based gel, containing chelated Fe^{3+}, in patients undergoing resection of the colon or rectum had to be discontinued early owing to the high rate of anastomotic leak in the treatment group.[51] As mentioned in the section on GI healing, serosal healing is vital to leak-free healing and interference with serosal migration and function is most likely responsible for the poor results.

Clinically, these barriers lead to an overall reduction in adhesion formation. Although the scoring systems and results vary, there does exist a role for using preventive devices. The only other remark is that although adhesion formation may be drastically reduced (either in number or severity), it is not completely abrogated, which many argue should be the goal of adhesion prevention.

REFERENCES

1. Gosain A, DiPietro LA. Aging and wound healing. World J Surg 2004;28(3):321–6.
2. Guo S, DiPietro LA. Factors affecting wound healing. J Dent Res 2010;89(3): 219–29.
3. Greenhalgh DG. The role of apoptosis in wound healing. Int J Biochem Cell Biol 1998;30(9):1019–30.
4. Singer AJ, Clark RA. Cutaneous wound healing. N Engl J Med 1999;341(10): 738–46.
5. Thompson SK, Chang EY, Jobe BA. Clinical review: healing in gastrointestinal anastomoses, part I. Microsurgery 2006;26(3):131–6.
6. Graham MF, Blomquist P, Zederfeldt B. The alimentary canal. Wound healing: biochemical and clinical aspects. Philadelphia: WB Saunders; 1992. p. 433.
7. Ellison G. Wound healing in the gastrointestinal tract. Semin Vet Med Surg (Small Anim) 1989;4:287–93.
8. Halsted WS. Circular suture of the intestine: an experimental study. Am J Med Sci 1887;94:436–61.
9. Graham MF, Diegelmann RF, Elson CO, et al. Collagen content and types in the intestinal strictures of Crohn's disease. Gastroenterology 1988;94(2):257–65.
10. Sturm A, Dignass AU. Epithelial restitution and wound healing in inflammatory bowel disease. World J Gastroenterol 2008;14(3):348–53.
11. Kilicoglu SS, Kilicoglu B, Erdemli E. Ultrastructural view of colon anastomosis under propolis effect by transmission electron microscopy. World J Gastroenterol 2008;14(30):4763–70.
12. Witte MB, Barbul A. Repair of full-thickness bowel injury. Crit Care Med 2003; 31(8):S538–46.
13. Herrmann JB, Woodward SC, Pulaski EJ. Healing of colonic anastomoses in the rat. Surg Gynecol Obstet 1964;119:269–75.
14. Månsson P, Zhang X, Jeppsson B, et al. Anastomotic healing in the rat colon: comparison between a radiological method, breaking strength and bursting pressure. Int J Colorectal Dis 2002;17(6):420–5.
15. Brasken P. Healing of experimental colon anastomosis. Eur J Surg Suppl 1991; 566:1–51.
16. Hendriks T, Mastboom W. Healing of experimental intestinal anastomoses. Dis Colon Rectum 1990;33(10):891–901.
17. Jiborn H, Ahonen J, Zederfeldt B. Healing of experimental colonic anastomoses: I. Bursting strength of the colon after left colon resection and anastomosis. Am J Surg 1978;136(5):587–94.
18. Jiborn H, Ahonen J, Zederfeldt B. Healing of experimental colonic anastomoses: II. Breaking strength of the colon after left colon resection and anastomosis. Am J Surg 1978;136(5):595–9.

19. Nelsen TS, Anders CJ. Dynamic aspects of small intestinal rupture with special consideration of anastomotic strength. Arch Surg 1966;93(2):309–14.
20. Granger DN, Hollwarth ME, Parks DA. Ischemia-reperfusion injury: role of oxygen-derived free radicals. Acta Physiol Scand Suppl 1986;548:47–63.
21. Mallick IH, Yang W, Winslet MC, et al. Ischemia-reperfusion injury of the intestine and protective strategies against injury. Dig Dis Sci 2004;49(9):1359–77.
22. Kologlu M, Yorganci K, Renda N, et al. Effect of local and remote ischemia-reperfusion injury on healing of colonic anastomoses. Surgery 2000;128(1):99–104.
23. Shandall A, Lowndes R, Young HL. Colonic anastomotic healing and oxygen tension. Br J Surg 1985;72(8):606–9.
24. Thornton FJ, Barbul A. Healing in the gastrointestinal tract. Surg Clin North Am 1997;77(3):549–73.
25. Kiyama T, Onda M, Tokunaga A, et al. Effect of early postoperative feeding on the healing of colonic anastomoses in the presence of intra-abdominal sepsis in rats. Dis Colon Rectum 2000;43(10):S54–8.
26. Dubay DA, Franz MG. Acute wound healing: the biology of acute wound failure. Surg Clin North Am 2003;83(3):463–81.
27. Ahrendt GM, Tantry US, Barbul A. Intra-abdominal sepsis impairs colonic reparative collagen synthesis. Am J Surg 1996;171(1):102–8.
28. Milsom JW, Senagore A, Walshaw RK, et al. Preoperative radiation therapy produces an early and persistent reduction in colorectal anastomotic blood flow. J Surg Res 1992;53(5):464–9.
29. Weiber S, Jiborn H, Zederfeldt B. Preoperative irradiation and colonic healing. Eur J Surg 1994;160(1):47–51.
30. Apostolidis SA, Michalopoulos AA, Hytiroglou PM, et al. Prevention of blood transfusion induced impairment of anastomotic healing by leucocyte depletion in rats. Eur J Surg 2000;166(7):562–7.
31. Barbul A, Knud-Hansen J, Wasserkrug HL, et al. Interleukin-2 enhances wound healing in rats. J Surg Res 1986;40(4):315–9.
32. O'Dwyer PJ, Conway W, McDermott EW, et al. Effect of mechanical bowel preparation on anastomotic integrity following low anterior resection in dogs. Br J Surg 1989;76(7):756–8.
33. Schein M, Assalia A, Eldar S, et al. Is mechanical bowel preparation necessary before primary colonic anastomosis? An experimental study. Dis Colon Rectum 1995;38(7):749–52 [discussion: 752–4].
34. Zmora O, Mahajna A, Bar-Zakai B, et al. Colon and rectal surgery without mechanical bowel preparation: a randomized prospective trial. Ann Surg 2003;237(3):363–7.
35. Mersin H, Bulut H, Berberoglu U. The effect of mechanical bowel preparation on colonic anastomotic healing: an experimental study. Acta Chir Belg 2006;106(1):59–62.
36. Kelly EE. Peritoneal adhesions, their symptomatology, pathology, and prevention. Cal State J Med 1904;2(1):9–11.
37. Buckman RF, Woods M, Sargent L, et al. A unifying pathogenetic mechanism in the etiology of intraperitoneal adhesions. J Surg Res 1976;20(1):1–5.
38. Ivarsson ML, Bergstrom M, Eriksson E, et al. Tissue markers as predictors of postoperative adhesions. Br J Surg 1998;85:1549–54.
39. Ray NF, Denton WG, Thamer M, et al. Abdominal adhesiolysis: inpatient care and expenditures in the United States in 1994. J Am Coll Surg 1998;186(1):1–9.
40. Barmparas G, Branco BC, Schnuriger B, et al. The incidence and risk factors of post-laparotomy adhesive small bowel obstruction. J Gastrointest Surg 2010. [Epub ahead of print].

41. Chegini N. TGF-β system: the principal profibrotic mediator of peritoneal adhesion formation. Semin Reprod Med 2008;26(4):298–312.

42. Tchernychev B, Furie B, Furie B. Peritoneal macrophages express both P-selectin and PSGL-1. J Cell Biol 2003;163(5):1145–55.

43. Ar'Rajab A, Dawidson I, Sentementes J, et al. Enhancement of peritoneal macrophages reduces postoperative peritoneal adhesion formation. J Surg Res 1995; 58:307–12.

44. Pados GA, Revroey P. Adhesions. Curr Opin Obstet Gynecol 1992;4:412.

45. Ellis H, Harrison W, Hugh TB. The healing of peritoneum under normal and pathological conditions. Br J Surg 1965;52:471.

46. Barbul A, Efron DT. Wound healing. In: Brunicardi FC, editor. Schwartz's principles of surgery. 9th edition. New York: McGraw Hill; 2009. p. 209–33.

47. Haney AF. Identification of macrophages at the site of peritoneal injury: evidence supporting a direct role for peritoneal macrophages in healing injured peritoneum. Fertil Steril 2000;73:988.

48. Burnett SH, Beus BJ, Avdiushko R, et al. Development of peritoneal adhesions in macrophage depleted mice. J Surg Res 2006;131:296–301.

49. Saed G, Jiang Z, Diamond M, et al. The role of myeloperoxidase in the pathogenesis of postoperative adhesions. Wound Repair Regen 2009;17(4):531–9.

50. Rajab T, Wallwiener M, Planck C, et al. A direct comparison of seprafilm, adept, intercoat, and spraygel for adhesion prophylaxis. J Surg Res 2010;161(2):246–9.

51. Tang CL, Jayne DG, Seow-Choen F, et al. A randomized controlled trial of 0.5% ferric hyaluronate gel (Intergel) in the prevention of adhesions following abdominal surgery. Ann Surg 2006;243(4):449–55.

Active Wound Coverings: Bioengineered Skin and Dermal Substitutes

Markéta Límová, MD*

KEYWORDS

- Skin substitutes • Bioengineered skin • Extracellular matrix
- Allogeneic • Autologous

In the last several decades, there has been a tremendous increase in the development of new active wound coverings and bioengineered skin substitutes. Increased understanding of wound healing and the complex interactions of cells, extracellular matrix molecules, growth factors, and various signaling molecules brought new materials that optimized wound healing and minimized scarring; these developments overcame the biochemical difficulties of chronic wounds and the challenges of extensive wounding found with large body surface area burns. Research has shown that moist wound healing creates a more optimal healing environment,[1,2] and this knowledge led to the development of various occlusive synthetic dressings that improved the outcome and addressed the various issues of acute and chronic wound environments. These new synthetic polymer dressings (**Table 1**) have improved the outcome in many situations and slowly replaced the centuries-old standard of gauze-type dressings. They can maintain an ideal moist wound environment, help autolytic debridement, prevent infection, and speed up granulation and epithelialization.[3] However, they are not always able to correct the challenges of complex chronic wounds or extensive wounding of the skin with large body surface area epidermal loss.

In recent years, a wide array of biologically active materials and skin substitutes has been developed. Although an ideal skin substitute is not yet available (**Box 1**),[4,5] these products address the various challenges of wound healing. Some of these materials can be used as dressings that protect the wound from fluid loss and infection. Others are used as wound implants that help replace extracellular matrix molecules or deliver various growth factors in an attempt to optimize the first stages of healing, preparing the wound for skin grafting and permanent skin coverage. The most advanced are

The author has nothing to disclose
Department of Dermatology, University of California, San Francisco, San Francisco, CA, USA
* 1340 West Herndon Avenue, Suite 101, Fresno, CA 93711.
E-mail address: scrockett@minaretsmed.com

Surg Clin N Am 90 (2010) 1237–1255
doi:10.1016/j.suc.2010.08.004
0039-6109/10/$ – see front matter © 2010 Elsevier Inc. All rights reserved.

Table 1 Synthetic dressings	
Type	**Composition**
Films	Polyurethane membrane
Hydrocolloids	Polymer with carboxymethylcellulose
Hydrogels	Polyethylene oxide/acrylates/acrylamides and water
Foams	Polyurethane foam
Alginates and Hydrofibers	Calcium alginate fibers (mannuronic and glucuronic acids) carboxymethyl cellulose fibers
Composites	Combination of several dressing types
Interactive	Antimicrobials, extracellular matrix, and other components incorporated into various dressing types

membranes that contain biologically active materials and live cultured cells, allogeneic or autologous in origin; the membranes attempt to regenerate skin using fibroblasts and keratinocytes in a scaffolding that can be implanted into the wound and lead to a more normalized healing. A summary and examples of these materials is listed in **Table 2**.

EXTRACELLULAR MATRIX MATERIALS

Extracellular matrix (ECM) materials are the first type of dressings that help change the environment of the wound and essentially can be considered *active* within the wound. These materials do more than just maintain an ideal moist wound-healing environment

Box 1 Properties of an ideal skin substitute
Increase healing
Decrease pain
Are safe
Are cost-effective
Are nonallergenic/-antigenic/-toxic
Are easy to apply and remove
Are flexible
Are moisture-permeable
Provide an infection barrier
Are durable/resist shearing
Recreate epidermis and dermis
Provide long-term/permanent wound cover
Are easy to manufacture and store
Are easy to obtain/easily available
Have a long shelf life
Data from Shores JT, Gabriel A, Gupta S. Skin substitutes and alternatives: a review. Adv Skin Wound Care 2007;20:493–508; and Pruitt BA Jr, Levine NS. Characteristics and uses of biologic dressings and skin substitutes. Arch Surg 1984;119:312–22.

Table 2
Bioengineered skin substitutes

Tissue Origin	Product	Manufacturer	Structure
Xenograft	Permacol	Tissue Science Laboratories, Aldershot, United Kingdom	Porcine dermis
	EZ derm	Brennen Medical, LLC, St Paul, MN, USA	Porcine dermis with aldehyde cross-linked collagen
	Matriderm	Suwelack Skin and Health Care Ag, Billerbeck, Germany	Bovine collagen coated with elastin.
	Oasis	Healthpoint, Fort Worth, TX, USA	Porcine intestinal submucosa
Synthetic	Biobrane	UDL Laboratories, Inc, Rockford, IL, USA	Silicone and nylon mesh bilayer with bound porcine collagen
	Integra	Integra Life Science Corp, Plainsboro, NJ, USA	Silicone and collagen/GAG matrix bilayer
	AWBAT	Aubrey, Inc, Carlsbad, CA, USA	Porous silicone and nylon knit bilayer with porcine collagen peptides
	Hyalomatrix	Fidia Advanced Biopolymers, Abano Terme, Italy	Silicone and esterified hyaluronan scaffold bilayer
Allogeneic			
Acellular	Cadaveric	Several	Processed fresh allogeneic dermis
	AlloDerm	Life Cell, Branchburg, NJ, USA	Processed allogeneic dermis
	Graftjacket	Wright Medical Technologies, Arlington, TN, USA	Freeze-dried decellularized allogeneic dermis
	GammaGraft	Promethean LifeSciences, Pittsburg, PA, USA	Gamma-irradiated allogeneic dermis
Epidermis	StrataGraft	StrataGraft Corp, Madison, WI, USA	Dermis and stratified allogeneic keratinocytes
Dermis	Dermagraft/ TransCyte	Advanced BioHealing, Inc, La Jolla, CA, USA	Bioabsorbable polyglactin mesh with neonatal fibroblasts
	ICX-SKN	Intercytex, Ltd, Manchester, United Kingdom	Bilayer silicone and nylon/collagen with neonatal fibroblasts Allogeneic ECM and fibroblasts
Composite	Apligraf	Organogenesis, Inc, Canton, MA, USA	Neonatal keratinocytes on collagen matrix with neonatal fibroblasts
	OrCel	Forticell Bioscience, Inc, New York, NY, USA	Neonatal keratinocytes and bovine collagen sponge with neonatal fibroblasts
Autologous			
Epidermis	Epicel	Genzyme Tissue Repair Corp, Cambridge, MA, USA	Cultured autologous keratinocytes
	Laserskin	Fidia Advanced Biopolymers, Abano Terme, Italy	HA mesh with autologous keratinocytes
	EpiDex	Modex Therapeutics, Lausanne, Switzerland	Silicone dishes with autologous stem cells
	Cell Spray	Avita Medical, Woburn, MA, USA	Cultured autologous keratinocyte suspension
Dermis	Hyalograft 3D	Fidia Advanced Biopolymers, Abano Terme, Italy	HA mesh with autologous fibroblasts
Composite	Cultured skin substitute	Several	Autologous cultured keratinocytes and fibroblasts grown in and on collagen/GAG matrix

Abbreviations: AWBAT, Advanced wound bioengineered alternative tissue; ECM, Extracellular matrix; GAG, glycosaminoglycans; HA, Hyaluronic acid.

by absorbing excess fluid or donating moisture. These dressings can actively change the wound environment by helping dermal regeneration, absorbing bacterial chemical byproducts and destructive wound enzymes (matrix metalloproteinases [MMPs]). These proteolytic enzymes play a role in cell migration through the ECM and help remodel the wound in the inflammatory phase of healing. In chronic nonhealing wounds, these enzymes remain at high levels and seem to be responsible for the uncontrolled degradation of existing and new ECM components; consequently, the balance of the equation is in favor of degradation rather than tissue repair. High levels of MMPs have been shown in a wide variety of wounds and are believed to develop from multiple causes, including bioburden of the wound, presence of nonviable tissue, and repeat trauma.[3]

Dressings specifically designed for helping reduce the high levels of MMPs are composed of a mixture of collagen and oxidized regenerated cellulose or alginate fibers. When such a dressing is placed into the wound, it chemically binds the various metalloproteinase-type enzymes and inactivates them. These materials have been shown, seemingly, to protect local growth factors from degradation by the MMPs, and therefore growth factors can remain biologically active in the wound environment.[6] Examples of such a dressing are Promogran Wound Matrix, Prisma, and Fibracol Plus Collagen (Johnson and Johnson, New Brunswick, NJ, USA).

To aid dermal regeneration, other materials composed of collagen or hyaluronic acid from various animal sources are used in the wound and are available in various forms. This exogenous collagen is thought to be chemotactic for fibroblasts and macrophages and also may provide a temporary 3-dimensional (3D) scaffold to help with the ingrowth of tissue.[7,8] Examples of these types of materials are Permacol (Covidien, Dublin, Ireland), Medifill (Human BioSciences Inc, Gaithersburg, MD, USA), Skin Temp (Human BioSciences Inc, Gaithersburg, MD, USA), and Matriderm (Suwelack Skin and Health Care Ag, Billerbeck, Germany), which are made from bovine-derived collagen material, and Oasis Wound Matrix (Cook Biotech, West Lafayette, IN, USA), which is porcine-derived.

MatriDerm is a dermal implant made of native bovine collagen coated with elastin. This matrix results in a better reconstruction of the dermis than pure collagen matrices and allows the ingrowth of host fibroblasts and other cells to regenerate a dermis with properties closer to normal uninjured skin. In a clinical study of acute burns, MatriDerm combined with autologous grafting gave better results in terms of elasticity and vascularization than skin grafting alone.[9,10] Also, wound contraction was significantly less in wounds treated with MatriDerm. Long-term follow-up showed that fibronectin formation of the dermis reconstructed with MatriDerm was comparable to normal, uninjured skin.[11,12] MatriDerm also allows the clinician to simultaneously place an autologous split-thickness skin graft within the same procedure, which helps minimize the need for a second operation in burn surgery.[13,14] This facilitates patients' recovery and, overall, enhances the rehabilitation process.

Oasis Wound Matrix is derived from porcine intestinal submucosa and is indicated for various types of partial- and full-thickness wounds, such as burns as well as traumatic and various chronic ulcers. This natural scaffold, which contains native ECM and various growth factors, is incorporated and absorbed into the wound base.[15] In vivo studies have shown angiogenesis into the matrix.[16] Oasis Wound Matrix has been evaluated in a randomized controlled clinical trial in the treatment of venous leg ulcers, and after 12 weeks, 55% of patients were healed in the Oasis group and only 34%, in the control group.[17] This material has the advantage of being fairly inexpensive, having excellent shelf life, and being easy to use.

ACELLULAR SKIN REPLACEMENTS
Synthetic Bilayer Substitutes

Synthetic bilayer substitutes are materials that consist of a porous matrix, which contains collagen, hyaluronic acid, fibronectin or other extra cellular matrix proteins, and a thin layer of silicone, which helps protect the wound from moisture loss and infection. Examples include Biobrane (UDL Laboratories Inc, Rockford, IL, USA), AWBAT (advanced wound bioengineered alternative tissue; Aubrey Inc, Carlsbad, CA, USA), Integra Bilayer Matrix Wound Dressing (Integra Life Science Corporation, Plainsboro, NJ, USA), and Hyalomatrix (Fidia Advanced Biopolymers, Abano Terme, Italy).

Biobrane is a biosynthetic skin substitute that is a bilaminate membrane consisting of nylon mesh with covalently bound porcine type I collagen peptide and a thin layer of silicone.[18] When it is applied to a partial-thickness or freshly excised full-thickness wound, it adheres and provides a temporary skin barrier. As the wound heals, fibroblasts and capillaries grow under the bilayer skin substitute and regenerate tissue in the dermis. The silicone layer functions as an epidermis, and pores in the silicone material allow some fluid to escape. In fairly superficial wounds, such as split-thickness donor sites, the membrane binds to the wound and is gradually replaced by host epithelium from adnexae and wound edges. In full-thickness wounds, the material stimulates granulation tissue and prepares the bed for autologous grafting, although the silicone membrane and nylon mesh need to be removed before the procedure. Since its development in 1979, Biobrane has become the standard for temporary coverage of freshly excised burn wounds.[4]

AWBAT is built on similar principles to Biobrane but with some significant modifications. It is composed of a very thin, porous silicone membrane bound to a loosely knit nylon fabric, which is coated with a mixture of porcine collagen peptides.[19] These peptides are not covalently bound as in the case of Biobrane, which allows them to interact more quickly with fibrin in the wound and allows better acute adherence during the initial phase of wound closure. More uniform distribution of pores in the silicone layer allows better fluid and moisture permeability and decreases the development of seromas at the wound site. Since this material was approved, it has been modified to impart somewhat varying physical properties and can be used for more specific types of wounds. AWBAT-Plus, the latest addition, uses the same bilayer membrane, except that it contains 6 xenogenic peptide components to further enhance wound healing.[20]

Integra Dermal Regeneration Template is another bilayer matrix that provides a scaffold for dermal regeneration and temporary wound coverage. The dermal replacement layer consists of a porous matrix of fibers of cross-linked bovine collagen and chondroitin-6-sulfate manufactured with a controlled porosity and defined degradation rate.[21] The epidermal substitute layer is made of a synthetic polysiloxane polymer and functions to control moisture loss from the wound and provide protection from infection. The collagen dermal replacement layer serves as a scaffold for the infiltration of fibroblasts and various other cells during the healing process. Over time, the dermal layer of Integra is degraded, replaced by host tissue, and neodermis is regenerated from the template. After 2 to 3 weeks, the silicone layer can be removed and thin meshed autologous grafts can be applied.[22,23]

This material is best used as an immediate skin replacement for the treatment of deep partial- or full-thickness burns. It can provide immediate closure for freshly excised wounds and helps maintain wound homeostasis during the recovery process. The healing time of a thin epidermal autograft on Integra template neodermis was comparable to conventional autograft. The cosmetic results are better than with conventional meshed autograft. Also, donor sites for the autografts healed faster and allowed more cycles of reharvesting than conventional donor sites when covered with Integra.[24,25]

The median take of Integra was comparable to conventional autograft, which was 95% successful overall.[22] There have been no reports of rejection. Integra has similar problems to other synthetic bilayer materials, such as problems with initial wound adherence and fluid accumulation under the dressing.[26] Integra is indicated for reconstruction after scar contracture, chronic ulcers, acute surgical wounds, and various other applications.[21]

Future developments and modifications of ECM materials are likely to focus on delivery of antimicrobial agents, growth factors, and DNA to further enhance wound healing. Colonization of wounds with bacteria occurs quickly and leads to formation of bacterial biofilm, which is believed to lead to chronic infections and can contribute to the development of various diseases and chronicity of wounds.[27] Incorporation of silver, cadexomer iodine, and other antimicrobial agents into ECM materials may help prevent or delay wound colonization and biofilm formation. Doxycycline, an antibiotic and MMP inhibitor, has been incorporated into chitosan microspheres and would be useful incorporated into various wound coverings.[28,29] With advances in polymer chemistry, microencapsulation and nanofibrous scaffolds have been constructed that can release DNA or growth factors at a controlled rate and over a longer period without degradation by MMPs, thereby optimizing outcome.[30–32]

Allogeneic Acellular Substitutes

Human cadaver allograft has been the gold standard for temporary coverage after burn wound excision for decades and is the standard to which most bioengineered skin substitutes are compared. It has also been tried in other types of wounds, such as chronic ulcers.[33] Dermal allografts are available through several sources, and they consist of human cadaveric skin that is cryopreserved, lyophilized, and glycerolized to remove donor cellular, infectious, and antigenic materials. The remaining structure serves as a scaffolding or template for the ingrowth of host fibroblasts and vascular tissue and helps regenerate dermal tissue. However, barrier function of human cadaver allografts is not ideal, shelf life is limited, and contamination of cadaver skin and disease transmission pose risks[34,35]; these drawbacks have instigated a search for other acellular dermal allograft products.

A few of the commercially available acellular dermal substitutes include Alloderm (Life Cell Inc, Branchburg, NJ, USA), Graftjacket (Wright Medical Technologies Inc, Arlington, TN, USA), Neoform (Mentor Corporation, Santa Barbara, CA, USA), DermaMatrix (Synthes Inc, Westchester, PA, USA), and GammaGraft (Promethean LifeSciences, Pittsburg, PA, USA). These are human cadaveric dermal products that differ in the manufacturing and processing steps, which give slightly different properties to the resulting allograft. Each material is marketed for different types of wounds depending on its use in studies, ranging from use as a base at the time of autologous grafting to use in orthopedic surgery, chronic wounds, and other applications (**Fig. 1A–E**). As with all allogeneic process tissue, a slight risk of disease transmission exists, because some native DNA remains; however, no such incident has been reported for any of these materials as there had been with frozen cadaveric allograft.[36–40]

LIVING SKIN SUBSTITUTES
Allogeneic Cellular Bioengineered Tissue

Epidermal substitutes
StrataGraft (StrataGraft Corporation, Madison, WI, USA) is a living human skin substitute. It consists of a dermal component that is layered with a fully stratified

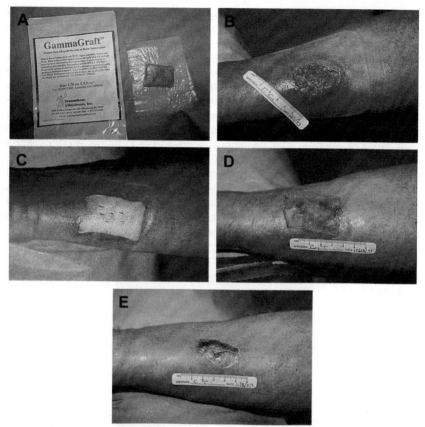

Fig. 1. (*A*) GammaGraft. (*B*) Debrided chronic ulcer. (*C*) Product placed on the wound. (*D*) Product adheres to wound base and provides a barrier one week later. (*E*) Two weeks later: note residual dried product partially debrided, exposing predominantly healed wound.

biologically functional allogeneic epidermis generated from neonatal immortalized keratinocytes. StrataGraft is pathogen-free and has tensile strength and barrier function comparable to that of intact human skin, including expression of host defense peptides, which, in turn, may help prevent infection.[41] This material is comparable to cadaver allograft for temporary management of skin defects. In various studies, there were no significant differences in autograft "take" between wound sites pretreated with StrataGraft and cadaveric allograft.[42]

Dermal substitutes

Dermagraft (Advanced BioHealing, Inc, La Jolla, CA, USA) is a cryopreserved human fibroblast-derived dermal substitute. It is manufactured from human newborn foreskin fibroblast cells seeded onto a bioabsorbable polyglactin mesh scaffold.[43] As the fibroblasts proliferate over the scaffold, they secrete various growth factors, cytokines, and ECM proteins and create a 3D human dermal substitute containing metabolically active cells.

The clinician receives the material frozen in a pouch, and after a simple thawing and rinsing procedure, it is ready to be used in the wound. The therapeutic properties are dependent on cell viability after cryopreservation, which is about 60%.[44] After implantation into the wound, the fibroblasts continue secreting various growth factors and may persist in the wound for several months, although eventually, they are replaced by host tissue.[45]

Dermagraft is currently indicated for the use and treatment of full-thickness diabetic foot ulcers lasting more than 6 weeks without muscle, tendon, joint capsule, or bone exposure, in which it has been shown to improve healing.[46,47] A US multicenter randomized controlled study showed complete closure at 12 weeks in 30% of the Dermagraft group compared with 18% in the control group.[48] Also, the Dermagraft group had significantly fewer ulcer-related adverse events. Dermagraft has also been used on other types of wounds, such as venous ulcers and fasciotomy wounds, although this is not Food and Drug Administration (FDA)-approved (**Fig. 2**A–D).[49,50]

A similar material is TransCyte (Advanced BioHealing Inc, La Jolla, CA, USA), which is a human fibroblast-derived temporary skin substitute consisting of a polymer silicone membrane and human neonatal fibroblast cells cultured onto a nylon mesh.[51,52] As the fibroblasts proliferate within the nylon mesh, they secrete various growth factors and ECM molecules, and the silicone membrane protects the wound. The material is cryopreserved, which leaves the various growth factors and ECM molecules intact. This membrane provides a transparent synthetic biologically active skin. Although multiple studies showed its advantages, TransCyte is not commercially available at this time.[53,54]

ICX-SKN is a single-layer dermal substitute comprised of collagen-based scaffolding populated with living fibroblasts. In early trials, ICX-SKN graft was successfully incorporated into the wound with complete revascularization.[55] This material is still undergoing clinical trials before becoming commercially available.

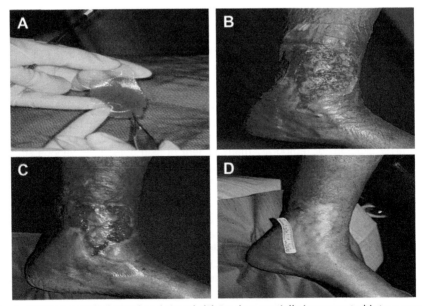

Fig. 2. (*A*) Dermagraft thawed and rinsed. (*B*) Product partially incorporated into a venous ulcer one week after placement. (*C*) Two weeks postplacement, wound showing areas of advancing epithelium. (*D*) Two months after initial treatment: wound closed.

Composite Skin Allografts

The most advanced commercially available allogeneic skin substitutes are bioengineered full-thickness human skin. They consist of a collagen scaffold with cultured fibroblasts and a layer of stratified cultured human keratinocytes. Although these products lack appendageal structures, vasculature, and rete ridges, the histology resembles normal skin (**Fig. 3**A, B). Two such products have been developed: Orcel (Forticell Bioscience, Inc, New York, NY, USA) and Apligraf (Organogenesis, Inc, Canton, MA, USA).

OrCel consists of a layer of cultured neonatal keratinocytes and a bovine collagen sponge with cultured neonatal fibroblasts. It is FDA-approved for the treatment of epidermolysis bullosa and split-thickness skin graft donor sites.[56–58] OrCel is cryopreserved, thus needing to be thawed and rinsed before placement into the wound. In clinical trials for venous insufficiency ulcerations, OrCel showed a statistically significant improvement in healing compared with the control group, and an application was filed with the FDA for the treatment of venous ulcers. Unfortunately, the company filed for bankruptcy before receiving approval, so this material is currently unavailable.

Apligraf is a composite bilayer product that consists of a layer of bovine type I collagen gel with cultured neonatal fibroblasts for its dermal component and a cornified epidermal layer of neonatal keratinocytes.[59,60] It is the only commercially available product of this type and is approved by the FDA for chronic venous ulcers lasting more than one month that have not responded to standard care and for full-thickness diabetic neuropathic foot ulcers lasting more than 3 weeks without exposed tendon, muscle, capsule, or bone. Patients treated with Apligraf experienced faster healing

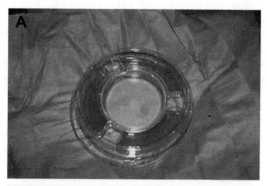

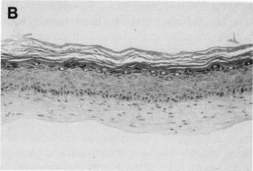

Fig. 3. Apligraft. (*A*) Appearance of product. (*B*) Microscopic appearance.

and decreased complication rate, thereby needing less medical follow-up.[61–63] In a large multicenter randomized controlled trial of nonhealing venous ulcers, Apligraf was found to be superior to standard compression therapy (63% vs 49%, respectively). Median time for ulcer closure was 61 days for the Apligraf patients compared with 181 days for the control group.[61,62] Apligraf was also shown to accelerate healing in diabetic neuropathic ulcers compared with standard therapy of moist gauze and off-loading.[63] After 12 weeks, 56% of the Apligraf patients were healed compared with 38% in the control group. There was also a lower rate of osteomyelitis and progression to amputation. Although the material is expensive, it has been shown to be cost-effective compared with standard therapy alone.[64,65] Apligraf has also been used to treat epidermolysis bullosa. In young pediatric patients, healing of the wound was observed in a few days, and they were able to maintain more normal mobility in their hands.[66–68]

Apligraf is an allogeneic product, although in many of the clinical trials, it seemed to be incorporated into the wound and engrafted. The transplanted cells were shown not to survive for a lengthy period of time and eventually were replaced by host cells.[69] Patients with epidermolysis bullosa were the exception, in whom the donor cells seemed to have survived for 6 months of the study period.[68] Apligraf has been used in various other clinical settings, such as acute surgical defects and split-thickness graft donor sites.[70–72]

Autologous Cultured Skin Replacements

For many years, the gold standard of permanent wound closure has been the use of autologous skin grafts. Unfortunately, in many patients with massive burns, the availability of donor sites is limited and also creates secondary wounds, which can lead to additional complications and scarring. In 1975, Rheinwald and Green[73] described a new way of culturing human keratinocytes, which allowed rapid, several thousand-fold expansion of the original skin sample, thereby creating a seemingly infinite supply of human epidermis.

This technique was first used in clinical practice in 1980 in an adult patient with burns.[74] The following year, it was used to treat 2 pediatric patients with burns who suffered 97% and 98% body surface area burns, which, without the substitute, would have been uniformly fatal.[75]

Since then, numerous patients have been treated with cultured epidermal autografts for burns and many other ulcerative conditions.[76–79] These grafts can provide permanent skin coverage in wounds with no other intrinsic sources of keratinocytes and can stimulate wound healing and re-epithelialization from the edges.

Serial cultivation of epidermal keratinocytes as described by Rheinwald and Green[73] leads to loss of cells that express HLA-DR markers.[80] Hence, it was thought that cultured allogeneic keratinocytes could be used, thereby avoiding a biopsy and delay in graft availability. Cultured allografts were used to treat various wounds without signs of rejection and with evidence of long-term persistence in the wound.[81–85] Ultimately, however, they are lost and are replaced with host epithelium. Also, the cosmetic and functional appearance of areas healed with cultured epithelial autografts is as good as, if not better than, areas treated with split-thickness skin grafts.[86] Cultured epithelial autografts are available as Epicel Cultured Epidermal Autograft (Genzyme Tissue Repair Corporation, Cambridge, MA, USA).[87] It was the first commercially available autologous bioengineered epidermal product available in the United States and is indicated for use in patients who have deep dermal or full-thickness burns covering more than 30% of body surface area. Epicel can be used alone or in conjunction with split-thickness autografts (**Fig. 4**).[87]

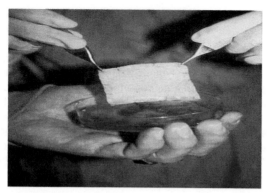

Fig. 4. EpiCel cultured epidermal autografts.

Cultured epithelial autografts, however, do present some challenges. They are quite fragile and susceptible to sheer injury and degradation by infection. The take can vary greatly from less than 20% to 100% depending on the condition of the wound bed and clinical technique. Another challenge with these grafts is the time taken to grow the epidermal sheets. Typically, the culturing process takes about 3 weeks, which poses challenges with patients' clinical care and temporary skin coverage issues. Although these grafts ultimately induce formation of a normal-appearing dermis, this process takes several years, so Epicel is currently used in conjunction with a dermal substitute. With ongoing research, other options may become available to clinicians that help address some of these issues.

Cell Spray (Avita Medical, Woburn, MA, USA) is cultured epithelial autograft suspension that is applied onto a clean wound bed using an aerosol applicator.[88] A small split-thickness donor biopsy is needed to start the process, and within about 5 days, viable preconfluent keratinocyte suspension can be produced. These cells proliferate and migrate within the wound bed; provide an even, confluent epidermal cell cover; promote healing; and optimize scar quality. Because burn wounds have a high risk of developing hypertrophic scarring, the longer a wound takes to heal, the higher the risk. Burn wounds that heal in less than 10 days have only a minimal risk of hypertrophy. Therefore, to provide early cell coverage onto such a wound is critical to cosmetic and functional scar outcomes. Cell Spray has been used in more than 1500 patients worldwide to treat various tissue injuries, and it can be used alone to treat partial-thickness injuries or with dermal reconstruction technology for deep dermal and full-thickness wounds.[89] The aerosolized method of application is much simpler, particularly in complex contour areas that are typically difficult to graft. Also, because keratinocytes retain the properties of the donor site, replacing skin with cell suspension from a matched donor site helps optimize outcome. Avita Medical has also developed the ReCell kit for the clinician. It is an autologous cell harvesting, processing, and delivery technology that prepares an autologous cell suspension within about 30 minutes. It can be used immediately on a wide variety of wounds and does not require specialized laboratory staff.

Another autologous keratinocyte graft previously reported is EpiDex (Modex Therapeutics, Lausanne, Switzerland). EpiDex is a cultured epidermal skin equivalent that is grown from hair follicle outer root sheath stem cells.[90] After a small amount of hair is plucked, the outer root sheath cells are grown in a coculture process designed to result in the formation of fully differentiated epidermis, mounted on silicone disks to facilitate handling. These disks are then applied onto the wound surface.

The rapidly dividing epidermal cells expand to cover the lesion.[91] The culturing process takes several weeks but has the advantage that no skin biopsy is required. This method has been used with success on various wounds, but additional larger controlled randomized studies are needed.[92–94] EpiDex is not available at this time.

Laserskin (Fidia Advanced Biopolymers, Abano Terme, Italy) is an epidermal autograft of cultured keratinocytes on a microperforated esterified hyaluronic acid. It has been used alone and in combination with autologous fibroblasts cultured on a hyaluronic acid matrix (Hyalograft 3D), making it the first full-thickness autologous skin replacement. Laserskin has been used on a wide variety of wounds with success; however, these studies were mainly retrospective and not controlled, so more evaluation is needed.[95–98] Laserskin and Hyalograft are not currently available in the United States.

FUTURE DIRECTIONS

Future research and development in the area of bioengineered skin substitutes is most likely to focus on improving full-thickness skin replacements; modifying culturing techniques; delivering growth factors, DNA and microRNA (miRNA); and improving full-thickness autologous skin substitutes.

Since the initial publication by Rheinwald and Green,[73] most skin cell culturing techniques have involved the use of bovine or porcine compounds and allogeneic or xenogeneic cells. Although minimal, these do pose some small risk of disease transmission, allergic reaction, and graft rejection. Recently, xenobiotic-free culture of human keratinocytes has been reported, including the use of autologous plasma as a scaffold for completely autologous bioengineered skin.[99–102]

Another area of potential future research and development is the delivery of pharmacologically active materials on cells into the wound, thereby modifying the wound environment.[103] The production of all tissue engineered skin substitutes involves combining cells, ECM, and cytokines in a bioreactor. ECM is necessary in order for certain cells to carry out their function and to activate or alter cytokine activity which in turn modifies the ECM. Fibroblast function and gene expression differs depending on body site, origin, and location in the dermis as well as culturing conditions.[104,105] This had been previously observed with oral epithelial cells and skin keratinocytes (author's observation[106]); therefore, the selection of the donor biopsy may allow the development of a skin substitute with particular properties suitable for certain body-site locations.

Discovery of miRNAs and their ability to regulate specific biologic functions has emerged as a particularly promising new area in wound research. It seems that miRNAs play a significant role in angiogenesis and other aspects of cell biology, and they might be used in wound healing to improve the wound base and increase graft take. An excellent review on this topic has been published by Sen.[107] Gene therapy is also an interesting area of potential development. Allogeneic cells can be genetically modified, cultured, and cryopreserved, then used when needed. They persist in the wound for some time but eventually are replaced by host cells, thereby minimizing long-term risks.[108]

Thicker dermal substitutes give better cosmetic outcome in terms of healing and hypertrophic scar formation; however, their major drawback is the length of time to complete revascularization and potential graft loss. Supplying a dermal substitute that already has a capillary network would increase take and improve outcome.[109–111] Endothelialized human reconstructed skin has been created by using a porous scaffold and coculturing fibroblasts and endothelial cells. This construct, over time, creates a 3D network of capillarylike structures within the reconstructed tissue.[110] When this material is transplanted into the wound, the preformed capillarylike structures connect with the host's vasculature within a few days. Such a material made using autologous cells would accomplish permanent replacement of dermis in the wound and should improve the outcome by achieving functionally better and more cosmetically pleasing skin.

Several groups have developed cultured, full-thickness, bioengineered autologous skin, although these materials are still early in their development. Cultured skin substitute developed at the University of Cincinnati is made by culturing autologous keratinocytes and fibroblasts with a collagen/glycosaminoglycans matrix. The results in burn patients were comparable to split-thickness skin grafts.[112] A Phase 2 randomized study of cultured skin substitutes versus split thickness skin grafts in patients with severe burn injuries is currently ongoing.[113]

A similar material was developed at VU Medical Center, Amsterdam, Netherlands, constructed from 3-mm punch biopsies and separate culturing of epidermis and dermis initially and lastly, allowing fibroblast migration into the dermal equivalent. The results in chronic ulcers were quite promising.[114]

Hopefully, the next few years will see a near-perfect skin substitute developed— a completely autologous, endothelialized, bioengineered skin that contains melanocytes, hair follicles, sweat, and sebaceous glands as well as adult stem cells that will be durable and cosmetically indistinguishable from normal skin.

REFERENCES

1. Winter GD. Formation of scab and the rate of epithelialization of superficial wounds in the skin of the young domestic pig. Nature 1962;193:293–4.
2. Hinman CD, Maibach HI. Effect of air exposure and occlusion on experimental human skin wounds. Nature 1963;200:377–8.
3. Ovington L. The art and science of wound dressings in the twenty-first century. In: Falabella A, Kirsner R, editors. Wound healing, 45. Boca Raton (FL): Taylor & Francis; 2005. p. 587–98.
4. Shores JT, Gabriel A, Gupta S. Skin substitutes and alternatives: a review. Adv Skin Wound Care 2007;20:493–508.
5. Pruitt BA Jr, Levine NS. Characteristics and uses of biologic dressings and skin substitutes. Arch Surg 1984;119:312–22.
6. Cullen B, Watt PW, Lundqvist C, et al. The role of oxidised regenerated cellulose/collagen in chronic wound repair and its potential mechanism of action. Int J Biochem Cell Biol 2002;34:1544–56.
7. Mian M, Beghe F, Mian E. Collagen as a pharmacological approach in wound healing. Int J Tissue React 1992;14:S1–9.
8. Harper C. Permacol: clinical experience with a new biomaterial. Hosp Med 2001;62:90–5.
9. Haslik W, Kamolz L-P, Nathschlager G, et al. First experiences with the collagen-elastin matrix Matriderm as a dermal substitute in severe burn injuries of the hand. Burns 2007;33:364–8.
10. Ryssel H, Gazyakan E, Germann G, et al. The use of Matriderm in early excision and simultaneous autologous skin grafting in burns – a pilot study. Burns 2008; 34:93–7.
11. van Zuijlen PP, Lamme EN, van Galen MJ, et al. Long term results of a clinical trial on dermal substitution. A light microscopy and Fourier analysis based evaluation. Burns 2002;28:151–60.

12. Haslik W, Kamolz LP, Manna F, et al. Management of full-thickness skin defects in the hand and wrist region: first long-term experiences with the dermal matrix Matriderm. J Plast Reconstr Aesthet Surg 2008;63:360–4.

13. van Zuijlen PP, van Trier AJ, Vloemans JF, et al. Graft survival and effectiveness of dermal substitution in burns and reconstructive surgery in a one-stage grafting model. Plast Reconstr Surg 2000;106:615–23.

14. Kolokythas P, Vogt PM, Boorboor P, et al. Simultaneous coverage of full thickness burn wounds with Matriderm dermal substitute and split thickness skin grafting. Burns 2007;33:S72.

15. Hodde JP, Ernst DM, Hiles MC. An investigation of the long-term bioactivity of endogenous growth factor in OASIS Wound Matrix. J Wound Care 2005;14:23–5.

16. Oasis Wound Matrix Web site. 2010. Available at: http://www.oasiswoundmatrix.com. Accessed May 23, 2010.

17. Mostow EN, Haraway GD, Dalsing M, et al. Effectiveness of an extracellular matrix graft (OASIS Wound Matrix) in the treatment of chronic leg ulcers: a randomized clinical trial. J Vasc Surg 2005;41:837–43.

18. Biobrane: biocomposite temporary wound dressings. 2009. Available at: http://www.udllabs.com/burn_care/biobrane.aspx. Accessed May 23, 2010.

19. Aubrey Inc. Available at: http://www.aubreyinc.com/awbat.html. Accessed May 23, 2010.

20. Woodroof EA. The Search for an ideal temporary skin substitute: AWBAT. Eplasty 2009;9:95–104.

21. Integra Dermal Regeneration. Integra LifeSciences Corporate Web site. Available at: http://www.integra-ls.com/home/. Accessed May 23, 2010.

22. Stern R, McPherson M, Longaker MT. Histologic study of artificial skin used in the treatment of full thickness thermal injury. J Burn Care Rehabil 1990;11:7–13.

23. Heimbach D, Luteman A, Burke JF, et al. Artificial dermis for major burns: a multi-center randomized clinical trial. Ann Surg 1988;S208:313–20.

24. Fitton AR, Drew P, Dickson WA. The use of a bilaminate artificial skin substitute (Integra) in acute resurfacing of burns: an early experience. Br J Plast Surg 2001;54:208–12.

25. Klein MB, Engrav LH, Holmes JH, et al. Management of facial burns with a collagen/glycosaminoglycan skin substitute-prospective experience with 12 consecutive patients with large, deep facial burns. Burns 2005;31:257–61.

26. Michaeli D, McPherson M. Immunologic study of artificial skin used in the treatment of thermal injuries. J Burn Care Rehabil 1990;11:21–6.

27. Phillips PL, Yan Q, Sampson E, et al. Effects of antimicrobial agents on an in vitro biofilm model of skin wounds. 6. In: Sen CK, editor. Advances in wound care, vol. 1. Columbus (OH): Liebert; 2010. p. 299–304.

28. Sapadin AN, Fleischmajer R. Tetracyclines: nonantibiotic properties and their clinical implications. J Am Acad Dermatol 2006;54:258.

29. Shanmuganathana S, Shanumugasundarama N, Adhirajana N, et al. Preparation and characterization of chitosan microspheres for doxycycline delivery. Carbohydr Polym 2008;73:201.

30. Shea LD, Smiley E, Bonadio J, et al. DNA delivery from polymer matrices for tissue engineering. Nat Biotechnol 1999;17:551–4.

31. Murphy WL, Mooney DJ. Controlled delivery of inductive proteins, plasmid DNA and cells from tissue engineering matrices. J Periodontal Res 1999;34:413–9.

32. Luu YK, Kim K, Hsiao BS, et al. Development of a nanostructured DNA delivery scaffold via electrospinning of PLGA and PLA-PEG block copolymers. J Control Release 2003;89:341–53.

33. Snyder RJ, Simonson DA. Cadaveric allograft as adjunct therapy for nonhealing ulcers. J Foot Ankle Surg 1999;38:93–101.

34. Barnett JR, McCauley RL, Schutzler S, et al. Cadaver donor discards secondary to serology. J Burn Care Rehabil 2001;22:124–7.

35. Mathur M, De A, Gore M. Microbiological assessment of cadaver skin grafts received in a Skin Bank. Burns 2008;35:104–6.

36. Wainwrigth DJ. Use of an acellular allograft dermal matrix (Alloderm) in the management of full-thickness burns. Burns 1995;21:243–8.

37. Munster AM, Smith-Meek M, Shalom A. Acellular allograft dermal matrix: immediate or delayed epidermal coverage? Burns 2001;27:150–3.

38. Brigido SA, Boc SF, Lopex RC. Effective management of major lower extremity wounds using an acellular regenerative tissue matrix: a pilot study. Orthopedics 2004;S27:145–9.

39. Rosales MA, Bruntz M, Armstrong DG. Gamma-irradiated human skin allograft: a potential treatment of modality for lower extremity ulcers. Int Wound J 2004;1:201–6.

40. Onur R, Singla A. Solvent-dehydrated cadaveric dermis: a new allograft for pubovaginal sling surgery. Int J Urol 2005;12:801–5.

41. Supp DM, Karpinski AC, Boyce ST. Expression of human beta-defensins HBD-1, HBD-2, and HBD-3 in cultured keratinocytes and skin substitutes. Burns 2004; 30:643–8.

42. Schurr MJ, Foster KN, Centanni JM, et al. Phase I/II clinical evaluation of StrataGraft: a consistent, pathogen-free human skin substitute. J Trauma 2009;66:866–74.

43. Dermagraft Web site. 2009. Available at: http://www.dermagraft.com/. Accessed May 23, 2010.

44. Mansbridge J, Liu K, Patch R, et al. Three-dimensional fibroblast culture implant for the treatment of diabetic foot ulcers: metabolic activity and therapeutic range. Tissue Eng 1998;4:403–14.

45. Harding KG, Moore K, Phillips TJ. Wound chronicity and fibroblast senescence-implications for treatment. Int Wound J 2005;2:364–8.

46. Gentzkow G, Jensen J, Pollak R, et al. Improved healing of diabetic foot ulcers after grafting with a living human dermal replacement. Wounds 1999;11:77–84.

47. Gentzkow GD, Iwasaki S, Hershon K, et al. Use of dermagraft, a cultured human dermis, to treat diabetic foot ulcers. Diabetes Care 1996;19:350–4.

48. Marston WA, Hanft J, Norwood P, et al. The efficacy and safety of Dermagraft in improving the healing of chronic diabetic foot ulcers: results of a prospective randomized trial. Diabetes Care 2003;26:1701–5.

49. Omar AA, Mavor AI, Jones AM, et al. Treatment of venous leg ulcers with Dermagraft. Eur J Vasc Endovasc Surg 2004;27:666–72.

50. Omar AA, Mavor AI, Homer-Vanniasinkam S. Evaluation of dermagraft as an alternative to grafting for open fasciotomy wounds. J Wound Care 2002;11:96–7.

51. TransCyte human fibroblast-derived temporary skin; Web site. Advanced Bio-Healing Inc. 2010. Available at: http://transcyte.com/. Accessed May 23, 2010.

52. Bello YM, Falabella AF, Eaglstein WH. Tissue-engineered skin. Current status in wound healing. Am J Clin Dermatol 2001;2:305–13.

53. Purdue GF, Hunt JL, Still JM Jr, et al. A multicenter clinical trial of a biosynthetic skin replacement, Dermagraft-TC, compared with cryopreserved human cadaver skin for temporary coverage of excised burn wounds. J Burn Care Rehabil 1997;18:52–7.

54. Kumar RJ, Kimble RM, Boots R, et al. Treatment of partial-thickness burns: a prospective, randomized trial using TransCyte. ANZ J Surg 2004;74:622–6.

55. Boyd M, Flasza M, Johnson PA, et al. Integration and persistence of an investigational human living skin equivalent (ICX-SKN) in human surgical wounds. Regen Med 2007;2:369–76.

56. Still J, Glat P, Silverstein P, et al. The use of a collagen sponge/living cell composite material to treat donor sites in burn patients. Burns 2003;29:837–41.

57. Sibbald RG, Zuker R, Coutts P, et al. Using a dermal skin substitute in the treatment of chronic wounds secondary to recessive dystrophic epidermolysis bullosa: a case series. Ostomy Wound Manage 2005;51:22–46.

58. Hasegawa T, Suga Y, Mizoguchi M, et al. Clinical trial of allogeneic cultured dermal substitute for the treatment of intractable skin ulcers in 3 patients with recessive dystrophic epidermolysis bullosa. J Am Acad Dermatol 2004;50: 803–4.

59. Apligraf Web site. 2009. Available at: http://www.apligraf.com/professional/index.html. Accessed May 23, 2010.

60. Trent JF, Kirsner RS. Tissue engineered skin: Apligraf, a bi-layered living skin equivalent. Int J Clin Pract 1998;52:408–13.

61. Falanga V, Margolis D, Alvarez O, et al. Rapid healing of venous ulcers and lack of clinical rejection with an allogeneic cultured human skin equivalent. Arch Dermatol 1998;134:293–300.

62. Falanga V, Sabolinski M. A bilayered living skin construct (APLIGRAF) accelerates complete closure of hard-to-heal venous ulcers. Wound Repair Regen 1999;7:201–7.

63. Veves A, Falanga V, Armstrong DG, et al. Graftskin, a human skin equivalent, is effective in the management of noninfected neuropathic diabetic foot ulcers: a prospective randomized multicenter clinical trial. Diabetes Care 2001;24: 290–5.

64. Schonfeld WH, Villa KF, Fastenau JM, et al. An economic assessment of Apligraf (Graftskin) for the treatment of hard-to-heal venous leg ulcers. Wound Repair Regen 2000;8:251–7.

65. Langer A, Rogowski W. Systematic review of economic evaluations of human cell-derived wound care products for the treatment of venous leg and diabetic foot ulcers. BMC Health Serv Res 2009;9:115.

66. Fivenson DP, Scherschun L, Cohen LV. Apligraf in the treatment of severe mitten deformity associated with recessive dystrophic epidermolysis bullosa. Plast Reconstr Surg 2003;112:584–8.

67. Falabella AF, Schachner LA, Valencia IC, et al. The use of tissue-engineered skin (Apligraf) to treat a newborn with epidermolysis bullosa. Arch Dermatol 1999; 135:1219–22.

68. Falabella AF, Valencia IC, Eaglstein WH, et al. Tissue-engineered skin (Apligraf) in the healing of patients with epidermolysis bullosa wounds. Arch Dermatol 2000;136:1225–30.

69. Phillips TJ, Manzoor J, Rojas A, et al. The longevity of a bilayered skin substitute after application to venous ulcers. Arch Dermatol 2002;138:1079–81.

70. Muhart M, McFalls S, Kirsner RS, et al. Behavior of tissue-engineered skin: a comparison of a living skin equivalent, autograft, and occlusive dressing in human donor sites. Arch Dermatol 1999;135:913–8.

71. Waymack P, Duff RG, Sabolinski M. The effect of a tissue engineered bilayered living skin analog, over meshed split-thickness autografts on the healing of excised burn wounds. Burns 2000;26:609–19.

72. Eaglstein WH, Alvarez OM, Auletta M, et al. Acute excisional wounds treated with a tissue-engineered skin (Apligraf). Dermatol Surg 1999;25:195–201.

73. Rheinwald JG, Green H. Serial cultivation of strains of human epidermal keratinocytes: the formation of keratinizing colonies from single cells. Cell 1975;6: 331–43.
74. O'Connor NE, Mulliken JB, Banks-Schlegel A, et al. Grafting of burns with cultured epithelium prepared from autologous epidermal cells. Lancet 1981;1:75–8.
75. Gallico GG III, O'Connor NE, Compton CC, et al. Permanent coverage of large burn wounds with autologous cultured human keratinocytes. N Engl J Med 1984;311:448–51.
76. Hefton JM, Caldwell D, Biozes DG, et al. Grafting of skin ulcers with cultured autologous epidermal cells. J Am Acad Dermatol 1986;14:399–405.
77. Carter DM, Lin AN, Varghese MC, et al. Treatment of junctional epidermolysis bullosa with epidermal autografts. J Am Acad Dermatol 1987;17:246–50.
78. Limova M, Mauro T. Treatment of pyoderma gangrenosum with cultured epithelial autografts. J Dermatol Surg Oncol 1994;20:833–6.
79. Limova M, Mauro T. Treatment of leg ulcers with cultured epithelial autografts: treatment protocol and five year experience. Wounds 1995;7:170–80.
80. Hefton JM, Amberson JB, Biozes DG, et al. Loss of HLA-DR expression by human epidermal cells after growth in culture. J Invest Dermatol 1984;83:48–50.
81. Thivolet J, Faure M, Demidem A, et al. Long-term survival and immunological tolerance of human epidermal allografts produced in culture. Transplantation 1986;42:274–80.
82. Thivolet J, Faure M, Demidem A, et al. Cultured human epidermal allografts are not rejected for a long period. Arch Dermatol Res 1986;278:252–4.
83. McGuire J, Birchall N, Cuono C, et al. Successful engraftment of allogeneic keratinocyte cultures in recessive dystrophic epidermolysis bullosa. Clin Res 1987; 35:702A.
84. De Luca M, Albanese E, Cancedda R, et al. Treatment of leg ulcers with cryopreserved allogeneic cultured epithelium: a multicenter study. Arch Dermatol 1992;128:633–8.
85. Teepe RGC, Roseeuw DI, Hermans J, et al. Randomized trial comparing cryopreserved cultured epidermal allografts with hydrocolloid dressings in healing chronic venous ulcers. J Am Acad Dermatol 1993;29:982–8.
86. Compton CC, Gill JM, Bradford DA, et al. Skin regenerated from cultured epithelial autografts on full-thickness burn wounds from 6 days to 5 years after grafting. A light, electron microscopic and immunohistochemical study. Lab Invest 1989;60:600–12.
87. Genzyme Web site. 2010. Available at: http://www.genzyme.com/. Genzyme Corporation. Accessed May 23, 2010.
88. Avita Medical Web site. Available at: http://www.avitamedical.com/. Accessed May 26, 2010.
89. Wood FM. Clinical potential of autologous epithelial suspension. Wounds 2003; 15:16–22.
90. Globe Newswire Web site. Modex Updates on Internal Programs: EpiDex and BioDelivery. Available at: http://www.globenewswire.com/newsroom/news. html?d=17715. Accessed June 4, 2010.
91. Limova M. Cultured skin substitutes. In: Falabella A, Kirsner R, editors. Wound healing, 42. Boca Raton (FL): Taylor & Francis; 2005. p. 550.
92. Tausche AK, Skaria M, Böhlen L, et al. An autologous epidermal equivalent tissue-engineered from follicular outer root sheath keratinocytes is as effective as split-thickness skin autograft in recalcitrant vascular leg ulcers. Wound Repair Regen 2003;11:248–52.

93. Hafner J, Kühne A, Trüeb RM. Successful grafting with EpiDex in pyoderma gangrenosum. Dermatology 2006;212:258–9.
94. Renner R, Harth W, Simon JC. Transplantation of chronic wounds with epidermal sheets derived from autologous hair follicles – the Leipzig experience. Int Wound J 2009;6:226–32.
95. Lam PK, Chan ES, To EW, et al. Development and evaluation of a new composite Laserskin graft. J Trauma 1999;47:918–22.
96. Lobmann R, Pittasch D, Mühlen I, et al. Autologous human keratinocytes cultured on membranes composed of benzyl ester of hyaluronic acid for grafting in nonhealing diabetic foot lesions: a pilot study. J Diabetes Complications 2003;17:199–204.
97. Uccioli L. A clinical investigation on the characteristics and outcomes of treating chronic lower extremity wounds using the tissuetech autograft system. Int J Low Extrem Wounds 2003;2:140–51.
98. Myers SR, Partha VN, Soranzo C, et al. Hyalomatrix: a temporary epidermal barrier, hyaluronan delivery, and neodermis induction system for keratinocyte stem cell therapy. Tissue Eng 2007;13:2733–41.
99. Sun T, Higham M, Layton C, et al. Developments in xenobiotic-free culture of human keratinocytes for clinical use. Wound Repair Regen 2004;12:626.
100. Coolen NA, Ulrich MMW, Middelkoop E. Future perspectives of tissue-engineered skin: xenobiotic-free culture systems. In: Sen CK, editor, Advances in wound care, 9. vol. 1. Columbus (OH): Liebert; 2010. p. 432–7.
101. Bullock AJ, Higham MC, MacNeil S. Use of human fibroblasts in the development of a xenobiotic-free culture and delivery system for human keratinocytes. Tissue Eng 2006;12:245–55.
102. Llames SG, Del Rio M, Larcher F, et al. Human plasma as a dermal scaffold for the generation of a completely autologous bioengineered skin. Transplantation 2004;77:350–5.
103. van Winterswijk PJ, Nout E. Tissue engineering and wound healing: an overview of the past, present, and future. Wounds 2007;19:277–84.
104. Chipev CC, Simon M. Phenotypic differences between dermal fibroblasts from different body sites determine their responses to tension and TFG β1. BMC Dermatol 2002;2:13.
105. Rennekampff HO, Xu W, Rodemann HP. Fibroblast subsets for skin substitute engineering. In: Sen CK, editor, Advances in wound care, 70. vol. 1. Columbus (OH): Liebert; 2010. p. 419–24.
106. De Luca M, Albanese E, Megna M, et al. Evidence that human oral epithelium reconstituted in vitro and transplanted onto patients with defects in the oral mucosa retains properties of the original donor site. Transplantation 1990;50:454–9.
107. Sen CK. Tiny new genes called microRNAs regulate blood vessel formation. In: Sen CK, editor. Advances in wound care, 7. vol. 1. Columbus (OH): Liebert; 2010. p. 353–8.
108. Koyama T, Aflaki P, Vranckx JJ, et al. Gene delivery to wounds using allogenic keratinocytes. In: Sen CK, editor. Advances in wound care, 8. vol. 1. Columbus (OH): Liebert; 2010. p. 382–7.
109. Schechner JS, Crane SK, Wang F, et al. Engraftment of a vascularized human skin equivalent. FASEB J 2003;17:2250–6.
110. Li WW, Talcott KE, Zhai AW, et al. The role of therapeutic angiogenesis in tissue repair and regeneration. Adv Skin Wound Care 2005;18:491.

111. Berthod F, Germain L, Pouliot R, et al. How to achieve early vascularization of tissue-engineered skin substitutes. In: Sen CK, editor. Advances in wound care, vol. 1. Columbus (OH): Liebert; 2010. p. 445–50.

112. Boyce ST, Kagan RJ, Greenhalgh DG, et al. Cultured skin substitutes reduce requirements for harvesting of skin autograft for closure of excised, full-thickness burns. J Trauma 2006;60:821–9.

113. Clinical Trials Web site. 2005. Available at: http://clinicaltrials.gov/ct2/show/NCT00004413. Accessed May 23, 2010.

114. Gibbs S, van den Hoogenband HM, Kirtschig G, et al. Autologous full-thickness skin substitute for healing chronic wounds. Br J Dermatol 2006;155:267–74.

Index

Note: Page numbers of article titles are in **boldface** type.

A

Acellular skin replacements, in wound coverings, 1241–1242
Active wound coverings, **1237–1255.** See also specific types.
    acellular skin replacements, 1241–1242
    allogeneic acellular substitutes, 1242
    allogeneic cellular bioengineered tissue, 1242–1244
    autologous cultured skin replacements, 1246–1248
    composite skin allografts, 1245–1246
    dermal substitutes, 1243–1244
    described, 1237–1238
    ECM materials, 1238–1240
    epidermal substitutes, 1242–1243
    future directions in, 1248–1249
    skin substitutes, living, 1242–1248
    synthetic bilayer substitutes, 1241–1242
    synthetic dressings, 1238
Allogeneic acellular substitutes, in wound coverings, 1242
Allogeneic cellular bioengineered tissue, in wound coverings, 1242–1244
Allograft(s), composite skin, in wound coverings, 1245–1246
Antibiotic(s)
    in biofilm eradication, 1154–1155
    in complex wound management, 1185–1186
Autologous cultured skin replacements, in wound coverings, 1246–1248

B

Biofilm
    bio-ecology of, 1149–1150
    characterization of, 1150–1152
    eradication of, 1152–1155
        antibiofilm agents in, 1155
        antibiotics in, 1154–1155
        chemical debridement in, 1153–1154
        mechanical debridement in, 1152–1153
        wound dressings in, 1153
    evaluation of
        direct observations in, 1151
        molecular techniques in, 1151–1152
    lifestyle of, 1148–1149
    protein upregulation and, 1150
    unique physiology of, 1149
    virulence and, 1150
    wound healing effects of, **1147–1160.** See also *Wound healing.*

Surg Clin N Am 90 (2010) 1257–1262
doi:10.1016/S0039-6109(10)00140-4
0039-6109/10/$ – see front matter © 2010 Elsevier Inc. All rights reserved.

surgical.theclinics.com

Moving?

Make sure your subscription moves with you!

To notify us of your new address, find your **Clinics Account Number** (located on your mailing label above your name), and contact customer service at:

Email: journalscustomerservice-usa@elsevier.com

800-654-2452 (subscribers in the U.S. & Canada)
314-447-8871 (subscribers outside of the U.S. & Canada)

Fax number: 314-447-8029

Elsevier Health Sciences Division
Subscription Customer Service
3251 Riverport Lane
Maryland Heights, MO 63043

*To ensure uninterrupted delivery of your subscription,
please notify us at least 4 weeks in advance of move.

Printed and bound by CPI Group (UK) Ltd, Croydon, CR0 4YY

03/10/2024

01040448-0013